PRAISE FOR

MW00366885

I LOVE this radically transformative book!!! As someone who
lives with daily chronic pain from CRPS, I can say *Unhackable
Soul* is a roadmap to reclaim your joy and reignite the light
within you despite pain! Maureen's authentic storytelling
illustrates how difficult experiences and deep wounds, both
mental and physical, are the very things that can gift us a deeper
power and resilience if we allow them. Maureen generously
brings us her personal journey and shares her formula for
moving through tremendous pain with grit and grace. Run,
don't walk, and grab this book if you live with any kind of pain!
—Amberly Lago
Podcast Host and Best-Selling
Author of *True Grit and Grace*,
TEDx Speaker, and Peak Performance Coach

Fantastically uplifting and encouraging from someone who
knows what it feels like to experience challenges and still live
life fully. Maureen's spirit shines through every page to speak
to you and pull you forward. Wonderful!
—Fiona Harrold
Best-Selling Author of *Be Your Own Life Coach*

Unhackable Soul is a resource and guide to achieving a fulfilling
life despite chronic pain. It offers a durable, livable alternative
to pharmacology and interventions. As a physician and surgeon
who has worked with chronic pain patients, I whole-heartedly
recommend this book for all who may live with chronic pain or
disability. It offers a sustainable path to healthy, balanced well-being
instead of a life of drugs, depression, and misery. In an era of
endemic opioids and dependency, it cracks in the light for the
pain sufferer on what can be for them an ever-darkening world.
—Dr Hugh A. Gelabert
Physician and Surgeon, UCLA School of Medicine

Maureen offers so many voices of comfort for the reader throughout *Unhackable Soul*. From comfort to knowing, practical advice and strategies, this book offers deep connection for many who may in some ways feel often isolated. Heartfelt and honest, this book will leave you hopeful. Be inspired by the thirty-year journey Maureen has been on, from which she shares an abundance of knowledge and practical advice to offer anyone feeling confused, depleted, or lost in the reality of chronic pain. Allow Maureen to hold your hand and be a comfort, and even a friend, through the deep work she offers in this book.

—Kamran Bedi
Author of *Your Mind is Your Home*,
PTSD and Anxiety Practitioner Utilising
Integral Eye Movement Therapy,
kamranbedi.com

As founder and CEO of the Burning Limb Foundation and one who is aware of the crucial role that mind and spirit play in individuals living with chronic pain disease, I highly recommend this book. Maureen's personal inspirational story and her step-by-step revitalizing daily elixir make this book a valuable go-to companion and guide for living well with pain and illness. Maureen's words incorporate ideas that are not just firmly rooted in truth but also come from a loving perspective that only one who has experienced debilitating illness intimately can bring. *Unhackable Soul* provides me with yet another tool when working with those who live with chronic illness and is a true blueprint for how not to just live but to thrive.

—Philip Robert
Founder/CEO of The Burning Limb Foundation

Unhackable Soul is emotionally compelling. It delivers an elixir that reaches deep into the heart, honoring and coaxing the reader to tap into the life within their own soul. Writing from the midst of her own experience, Maureen validates the temptation to retreat while modeling the choice to rise and embrace a life of joy. Full of grace, grit, and wisdom, *Unhackable Soul* is a must-read for anyone suffering chronic illness and pain.

—Danielle Bernock
Victorious Souls Podcast, Author of *Emerging With Wings: A True Story of Lies, Pain, And The LOVE that Heals*

Maureen's book is a testament to showing you have a choice in how you deal with a chronic condition. With chronic pain on the increase, this is a refreshing, holistic, and empowering guide to help people take back control and take back their lives.

—Dr Sohère Roked
UK GP and Functional Medicine and Hormone Doctor, Author of *The Tiredness Cure*

At last, a practical book on chronic pain by somebody who lives with and copes with way more than her fair share of it. I use one particular tip of Maureen's as a personal mantra to get me through my pain days. Open the book, read it, re-read it. Find yours. They're powerful.

—Ann Jackson
Invisible Pain Fighter and Special Needs Teacher

There are so many books out there about 'living your best life', but few have the realism, joy, and compassion that Maureen pours out of her heart and onto the pages of this book. As a young man who has battled Complex Regional Pain Syndrome for almost ten years, I find Maureen's words of wisdom and encouragement a true inspiration and blessing.

—Gabriel C. King

Throughout the book, Maureen gently takes readers by the hand and acts as a guide, nurturing at the readers' pace, giving them permission to be themselves. *Unhackable Soul* is both enriching and powerful, speaking directly to those living with a chronic illness or disability and equally speaking to those supporting the individuals—medically and personally. As a mother of a daughter who was diagnosed with cerebral palsy at thirteen months old and having subsequently developed a long-term health condition myself, I know one thing for sure—the description of your label does not define who you are as a human being. Live a limitless life your way—your past does not equal your future. *Unhackable Soul* is the perfect prescription to start your journey and live your best life.

—Sera Johnston
International Best-Selling Author, Health and
Mindset Coach, and Development Consultant:
Empowering Mothers Raising Children with Disabilities
Reclaim their Identity, Health, and Happiness

Maureen's elixir for self-healing and management of chronic pain and illness is a refreshing perspective in a world with prevalent addictions to pain medication. Based on her own personal history with chronic and severe pain and illness, these techniques come from decades of experience with her own journey. With an invitation to dig deep inside yourself to discover the joy of living in spite of pain, she really does close the gap between retreating from life and rising to meet it where you are. This book gives you but a taste of how amazing this author is and how she has overcome.

—Tammy Green
Author of *Living Without Skin: Everything I
Never Knew About Fierce Vulnerability*

I have been a long-term warrior of chronic pain and chronic fatigue. My mantra for many years has been 'Fall down seven times, stand up eight', which is a Japanese proverb. I loved Maureen's book, and reading it made me feel more positive. It is easy to get dragged down when you are in chronic pain. There are lots of tips to help in the book. It's good, fantastic actually, to be reminded that 'I am not my physical body. I am not my self-limiting mind. I am the soul and spirit within. I am me.' Keep this book handy to dip into when you are not having your best day.

—Louise Scott

Maureen's realness immediately connects with and encourages those walking the path of chronic pain, rekindling joy, and shining light on otherwise dark days. This book truly makes a difference as her joy is contagious.

—Lori King
Proud Mom of a CRPS Warrior

Maureen writes with an immensely clear and resoundingly authentic voice that is combined with an unparalleled depth and breadth of personal experience and embodied wisdom to reach directly into the hearts and minds of her readers. Highly recommended.

—Julia McCutchen
Intuitive Coach, Mentor, and Author

UNHACKABLE
SOUL

Unhackable Soul

Rise Up, Feel Alive, and Live Well with Pain and Illness

The 30-Day Elixir for Reigniting the Light Within

Maureen Sharphouse

Based on *Unhackable*—
The *Wall Street Journal* and *USA Today* Best-Seller

UNHACKABLE
PRESS

Published by Unhackable Press
PO Box 43, Powell, OH 43065
www.UnhackableBook.com

Library of Congress Cataloguing: 2022903293

Paperback: 978-1-955164-06-1
Hardback: 978-1-955164-07-8
Ebook: 978-1-955164-08-5

Available in softcover, hardcover, e-book, and audiobook.

Scripture quotations from The Authorized (King James) Version. Rights in the Authorized Version in the United Kingdom are vested in the Crown. Reproduced by permission of the Crown's patentee, Cambridge University Press.

The information given in this book should not be treated as a substitute for professional medical advice; always consult a medical practitioner. Any use of information in this book is at the reader's discretion and risk. Neither the author nor the publisher can be held responsible for any loss, claim, or damage arising out of the use, or misuse, of the suggestions made, the failure to take medical advice, or for any material on third party websites.

To all who live with pain and illness,
this book is for you.

And to all my family, especially my
mother and my husband, Peter:
Your love keeps me strong.

DISCLAIMER

All the techniques and methods introduced and explored in this book can be used alongside medical treatment. They are not intended as a substitute. If you are experiencing undiagnosed pain and other symptoms you are concerned about, it is encouraged that, in addition to reading this book, you seek advice from a qualified medical practitioner or suitable therapist. Maureen Sharphouse is not a doctor or certified medical professional. She is a pain and illness patient, peer support advocate, an accredited and certified life coach and mentor, NLP Master Practitioner, writer, and speaker, putting to purpose what she has come to know to help others who are experiencing pain and illness. Her desire is to help readers enjoy greater joy and comfort in their lives, ignite and unleash the fire and passion of the soul and spirit within them, and live their best lives.

CONTENTS

PART THREE

RESTOKE

Part Four

Enliven

Part Five

Rise

FOREWORD

You know what it's like. You have big dreams and goals in life and a lengthy bucket list you want to achieve. You envision a happy life full of rewarding relationships and a successful career. You see yourself enjoying a never-ending love and zest for life. You make plans for your next challenge. Joy and fun await.

And then it happens. Your plans are interrupted. The trajectory of your life hits a roadblock.

One minute you are boldly sailing on course, enjoying life to the full, and the next moment all thoughts of a bright rewarding future and your dreams dissolve into the background.

Something knocks you off course. Life gets in the way. And whether the culprit is something you don't have full control of or it is the result of something you did, it can crush your spirit and leave you without hope.

In short, your soul becomes *hacked*—you find yourself 'alive' but mostly numb and dead on the inside.

You are about to read an insightful book from my friend Maureen Sharphouse. Even though we live on opposite sides of the globe and have yet to meet in person, she exudes Unhackable joy, enthusiasm, love, and passion for life. I would call her a 'soul on fire'! It is difficult to comprehend that she lives with a debilitating, progressive, incurable neurological illness, which due to its intensely severe and relentless high pain levels, is commonly known as 'the suicide disease'.

Maureen knows first-hand the roller coaster of emotions, difficulties, and challenges of living with ongoing pain and disability. She has experienced many pain crises and overwhelming dark moments. Nevertheless, over the last three and a half decades, Maureen has discovered a proven process to rise up, feel alive, and live well with pain and illness.

Today is your day to start the same process. As you read *Unhackable Soul* with an open mind and fully digest all this book offers, you too can take your best next step to a full life. Her 30-day elixir is enlightening, liberating, and powerful. Take your time. Don't race to the end. Consume it at a pace that is comfortable for you.

The insights, wisdom, and clarity you need are on every page— unpack each one and then go create a new story of your own!

With its empowering thirty daily missions, this book will guide you through new ways of thinking and inspire you to rise from within your circumstances.

If you are fed up living a life dictated by pain and illness and want to live a legacy you are proud of, this book is for you. Maureen will help you become an Unhackable Soul!

—Kary Oberbrunner
The Wall Street Journal and *USA Today* Best-Selling Author
of *Unhackable*
and CEO of Igniting Souls Publishing Agency

WELCOME:
A NOTE TO YOU—THE READER

This is your moment.
You are meant to be here.

—Herb Brook

Hello there. I am glad *Unhackable Soul* has found you, but I am sorry you are hurting. It's likely you picked up this book because you or someone you deeply care about lives with pain and illness. I am sorry for that pain.

I know it feels as though few people understand what it is like to live with the cruel mistress of pain 24/7. Pain can hack your soul, erode your spirit, and squeeze the joy right out of life. It can make you feel bitter. Given half a chance, pain will dictate the person you become. It shapes and colours how you spend each day as it determines what you feel you can and cannot do. Left unchecked, pain can send you spiralling down an ever-darkening hole where life becomes no more than an unfulfilling day-to-day existence. It tests your mental resilience. As dreams die and feelings of isolation set in, your perception of your self-worth diminishes.

I understand because, to date, I have lived with intractable neurological pain as my relentless companion for more than three decades of my life. I have travelled down many a dark tunnel of pain and been overwhelmed by tsunamis of despair. Pain has dropped me to my knees at times and left me sobbing as I've pleaded for relief.

And yet, today, I feel more vibrantly alive than ever.

Through the years, I have learned that fighting the pain—doing all you can to deny or block it—does not help. Nor does letting it take the driver's seat of your life. And in terms of learning to live and enjoy life, neither of those coping strategies are helpful.

As difficult as it is to endure chronic pain and illness, you are not the only one who suffers. Family members, friends, and colleagues hurt for you also, even although they cannot fully comprehend what it is like to live with pain day in and day out.

Chronic pain is defined as pain lasting longer than twelve weeks despite medication, medical interventions, or treatment. Sadly, current research indicates that around 1.5 billion people[1] suffer from chronic pain. Around 50.2 million[2] adults in the USA (20.5 percent) experience it, with the estimated total value of lost productivity due to chronic pain being nearly $300 billion annually. In Europe, it affects around 20 percent[3] of people, with almost ten million[4] Britons suffering daily.

At the time of this book's writing, the world is facing the COVID-19 pandemic. With the ongoing debilitating symptoms and musculoskeletal pain that many people are experiencing following their initial recovery from the virus (referred to as 'long COVID'), sadly, pain and illness statistics are likely to get worse.

Medical professionals often offer little hope for healing or a cure when pain is chronic. Surgeries, specialised treatments, opioids, and medication intended to heal, alleviate, or block the pain frequently prove ineffective and come with unwanted side effects. Getting through each day for the pain sufferer becomes an ongoing challenge. Unrelenting pain taxes every aspect of life, ripping relationships apart, thwarting careers, dreams, and goals, draining finances, and stretching physical and emotional resources to their limits.

Chronic pain is a complete physical, mental, and emotional assault that can make you feel ashamed, upset, or disappointed with life—with yourself. But I want you to know this: You are not your pain and illness. Neither are you defined by any health condition, life events, circumstances, health labels, or ongoing challenges.

You are soul and spirit, not merely flesh; your physical body is simply the suit you wear and the vehicle you operate through whilst you are here on planet Earth in human form.

You are who you are within; you are who you choose to be.

This book does not promise you the tools for a miracle cure or fix. Nor can I promise you that instigating and fully embodying the practices and mindsets within these pages will bring about full physical healing. The mind–body connection is powerful, and it is imperative you understand how each interacts and impacts the other. Sometimes, however, despite what many mindset coaches or mind–body gurus teach, full healing at a physical, functional level is not always possible. That said, wellness is often about keeping your soul and spirit healthy, even when your physical body is injured, deteriorating, ageing, or impaired in some way. Living *well* happens when we develop an Unhackable Soul—the ability to see the beauty in imperfection and to rise, enriched by truth, and start each day anew.

How to Get the Most Out of This Book

Throughout this book, I will introduce new ways of thinking, practical and spiritual strategies, and ways of living that can help ignite a renewed enthusiasm and passion within you. The thirty daily missions I will share are the same steps I took to rise from the dark pit dug by pain and transform my quality of life. Today, my life is rooted in—and my soul is nourished by—these fundamental principles.

By applying what I share with you on this thirty-day journey, you will be doing all you can to aid your physical body's natural healing mechanisms by getting your soul and spirit, as well as your emotional, psychological, and mental state in their best condition. Only you can be your rescue, however, and you have to decide how much you will apply from the pages that follow.

Knowing all too well that living 24/7 with pain and illness can make it difficult to focus and concentrate for lengthy periods, I wrote *Unhackable Soul* with you in mind. You'll notice that there are no chapters, only days. You can digest the content one day at a time, or you may wish to read multiple days at a time.

I encourage you to read and apply the steps in this book at a pace that feels relaxed and comfortable to you. Answer the reflective questions, explore, and put into practice the strategies I share with you, and complete the daily 'Rise' simple assignments. See yourself as a work in progress. Meaningful and sustainable change takes time, so be understanding and patient; you do not need to implement everything I share with you immediately or all at once.

Above all, be gentle and kind to yourself. Living with pain and illness can be challenging at best and debilitating at worst. Use this book as fuel to nourish, guide, and support you on this journey to living well with pain and illness.

I have a story; you have a story. Our stories unite us. We are the same.

Maureen

THE DAY IT BEGAN

*Recognising that you are not where you want to be
is a starting point to begin changing your life.*

—Deborah Day

The morning of Wednesday, 27 November 2002 started much like any other day. Mike, my husband at that time, and our children shouted goodbye as they flew out the door for work and university. My care assistant, Irene, popped in briefly to help bathe and dress me and settle me in my usual chair in the front room next to the fireplace. She placed a cup of hot milky tea on the small table beside me. Looking through the window, I could see the day was still dark, although it was already after nine. It felt as though there had been no sun for years.

I picked up the television remote and flicked through the channels, but I had no appetite that morning for hearing about family breakdowns or watching home makeovers. Switching on the radio, a familiar song filled the room, 'Though it's darker than December, what's ahead is a different colour.' The hopeful words of the song *High* by Lighthouse Family had come to mean so much to me since I had become too ill to work some five years earlier. Usually, the song lifted my spirits, but that day, I shouted, 'You're lying! What's ahead isn't a different colour. For me, it's all the same.'

I looked around the room at the wheelchair by the door, the Zimmer walking frame next to me, and the boxes of painkillers on the coffee table. The small carriage clock on the mantelpiece chimed. It was 9:30 a.m., and it would be another nine or ten hours before any of my family would return home for a quick bite to eat and then likely head back out to meet friends for the evening. Loneliness and pain were my life, and I knew it might remain that way for the next thirty or forty years.

That morning, the horrible realisation hit me as if for the first time.

I saw my life spread out in front of me, day after day—hundreds and thousands of days of sitting there, waiting for my mother to visit and take me out in my wheelchair, waiting for carers to help me get bathed and dressed. . . .

Nothing would be different.

It would be the same for years to come.

With my whole body, I cried out, '*No!*'

No to the doctors, *no* to the hospitals, *no* to the carers, *no* to the pain, *no* to the financial worries—*no* to everything.

I was only forty-six years old. I felt I had not yet lived.

That moment, I saw myself clearly. Although I was breathing and my heart beat steadily within me, my soul and spirit had been hacked—something had gained unauthorized access to my life. Despite being physically alive, I felt dead.

The harsh realisation that I had lost all passion and joy was my catalyst for taking ownership of my life and redirecting the story I was living. In that standout moment, I committed to doing all I could to crack the darkness open and let the light of a better future start to stream back in. For five years, I had retreated deeper and deeper into the darkness of pain, loneliness, and despair. But that was not how I wanted to live. I wanted to rise up, feel alive, and live well despite my pain and illness. I wanted to reignite the light within me.

You must do the same.

RETREAT OR RISE: YOUR TIME IS NOW

You have a choice. Will you retreat to the side-lines of life and let your pain and illness dictate your quality of life? If you have had enough of living a life that does not feel as purposeful and rewarding as you would like, I encourage you to rise and thrive from within your circumstances.

You and I are ever-evolving souls. At any point, we can choose to say, 'Enough is enough; I am sick and tired of being sick and tired all the time. A life controlled by pain and illness is not how my story is going to end.'

That dark morning in my front room, I made the choice to rise. Today, although I still live with chronic pain, my soul, spirit, and mind are strong and vibrant. And as a result, my life is wholly different—it is much brighter and happier and no longer marked by feelings of numbness and isolation.

Are you ready to rise? Do you long to reignite fire in your soul and live a life fuelled by enthusiasm and purpose rather than dictated by pain?

I believe you can, and I am excited to come alongside you on this journey.

Let us begin. . . .

PART ONE

UNVEILING

*The Earth school is one of the most difficult in
the Universe: only the bravest souls sign up.*

—Dolores Cannon

DAY 1
FACE YOUR STORY

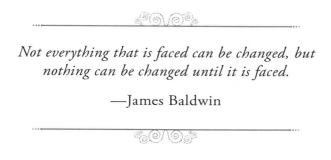

*Not everything that is faced can be changed, but
nothing can be changed until it is faced.*

—James Baldwin

Face

1. to confront and deal with or accept a difficult or
   unpleasant task, fact, or situation

2. to acknowledge and accept (facts, truth, etc.)

3. to accept the reality that a bad situation exists and
   try to deal with it

> —Definitions sourced from 1) Lexico Dictionaries,
> 2) YourDictionary, and
> 3) Macmillan Dictionary.

***In a Nutshell: To face is to realise and be ready to meet your
circumstances, truth, and facts.***

On the night of that pivotal day when I screamed 'enough is enough' to the life I was living, I went to bed feeling strong and powerful. A sense of excitement and purpose overcame me as I envisaged the possibility of a brighter future.

The next morning, I awoke feeling numb and weak once again. As I'd slept, my excitement had diminished along with my inner strength to fight for a more meaningful and joyful life. In truth, I felt stupid for having even considered change possible. I shuffled to the mirror where a hollow-eyed figure stared back at me. What on earth had I been thinking? I felt weak and childish and questioned my judgment, thinking that all that hope and enthusiasm were probably the result of overmedication. *How could I possibly have imagined anything other than a bleak future?*

I sat for a while, transfixed by the image in the mirror—and I felt horrified and uneasy. I hated *me* and what had become of me. I despised the downward spiral that had become my life. Seeing that pitiful figure staring back at me from the mirror was the sharp shake-up I needed. I saw that my happiness was *my* responsibility—it came down to no one else. If I was serious about crafting change in my life, I knew I had to *start somewhere.* So I rummaged around in the drawer in my dressing table, found some lip gloss, and for the first time in a long time, I put some on.

The simple act of putting on lip gloss may seem insignificant, but today, almost twenty years later, that moment stands out as a major turning point in my life. I realised that facing the reality of my circumstances and igniting a desire for a better life was never going to be enough on its own.

If I didn't take some positive action, my desire would remain only a wish and a dream. And what I have come to know is that even the smallest steps, when taken consistently, add up in time.

> IF I DIDN'T TAKE SOME POSITIVE ACTION, MY DESIRE WOULD REMAIN ONLY A WISH AND A DREAM.

ONE SMALL STEP

If you are not happy with the life you are currently living but do nothing to change it, you will only experience more of the same. Doing nothing while waiting on a golden day to miraculously transform your quality of life will leave you dwelling in your discomfort for an exceedingly long time.

You must *choose* to bring more heartfelt joy into your life and *take responsibility* for being the change you want to see in your world. Clinging to the darkness in your pain may inspire empathy, care, help, or support from others, but it will not encourage fresh opportunities for thinking anew about your circumstances—nor will it manifest a better life.

You *deserve* to be happy and experience success and joy in your life, irrespective of the pain or illness that accompanies you on life's journey. Dwelling in your discomfort and being the victim of it will never lead to your healing—in whatever form your physical, emotional, or psychological healing may come.

While it is important to work alongside doctors and medical professionals who understand your health condition, it is essential to recognise that medicine has its limitations. Surgeries, therapies, and prescription drugs can be helpful (and in some instances are vital to your well-being and survival), but medicine alone can never provide the complete answer to living well inside as well as out.

Know you are allowed to scream, grieve, or cry at times; you are allowed to shout and temporarily drop to your knees in despair. But you must not give up on life and especially not give up on *you!*

The path you must choose to walk may feel rough at times, however, you cannot wait for a day to feel 'better.' Don't wait for your mood to seemingly improve before you decide to say *enough is enough* and start crafting meaningful and positive change in your life.

Sitting back and doing nothing is not going to make for a better today, better tomorrow, better next week, or better next year.

Today is Day 1 of your elixir, and it's time to face your story the same way I did. Keep change simple and take small steps. Start by acknowledging current circumstances and who you are within those circumstances. This is the beginning of your story.

Keeping Things Simple: Do nothing now, nothing much changes. Crafting a brighter future comes down to you.

RISE: FACE YOUR STORY

When we deny the story, it defines us. When we own the story, we can write a brave new ending.

—Brené Brown

Positive change isn't created by ignoring or denying what is happening; it comes from being honest with yourself. Your first *Rise* assignment is to get real by facing the truth of who you are right now and how you live your life. Use this book as your safe place to take notes, make admissions, and identify how you want your life to change. Be open and honest with yourself.

Review the following questions and circle the answer that is most appropriate to you at this present time:

How often do I feel enthusiastic about my day when I wake up in the morning?

Never   Hardly Ever   Sometimes   Most of The Time   Always

How often do pain and illness dictate my day?

Never   Hardly Ever   Sometimes   Most of The Time   Always

How often do I allow myself to have fun and hear myself laughing?

Never   Hardly Ever   Sometimes   Most of The Time   Always

How often do I have a sense of fulfilment and contentment at the end of the day?

Never   Hardly Ever   Sometimes   Most of The Time   Always

How often do I feel that life is passing me by whilst everyone around me seems to be getting on and having success and fun?

Never   Hardly Ever   Sometimes   Most of The Time   Always

How often do I feel down about my circumstances, sad, depressed, or anxious?

Never   Hardly Ever   Sometimes   Most of The Time   Always

When I think about my future, how often do I envisage it as bright, exciting, meaningful, and rewarding?

Never   Hardly Ever   Sometimes   Most of The Time   Always

On a scale of 1 to 10 (10 being the highest), how happy do I currently feel?

1   2   3   4   5   6   7   8   9   10

Be proud. Opening your eyes to your current reality is not always easy. If your answers have left you feeling somewhat raw and vulnerable, I want you to know that is okay. After I had made my 'enough is enough' decision, I felt as though I had been catapulted naked into a swirling abyss. I had no idea what I needed to do to change my circumstances. Being clear and honest about my starting point empowered me to face my reality. The same will be true for you. Truth is the best possible place from which to craft positive change.

Congratulations! You have made a great first step! Now it's time to take your first small action.

Celebrate your honesty and courage by rewarding yourself with something that uplifts you or makes you feel good. It does not need to be big, demanding, or difficult. Remember, I put on a touch of lip gloss. Your small step can be as simple as making yourself a coffee, chatting on the phone to a friend, putting on a bright coloured shirt, listening to a piece of uplifting music, or sitting in your garden for a few minutes. When you have done that, breathe in renewed energy.

When you are ready, join me for Day 2.

DAY 2
SHED YOUR LABELS

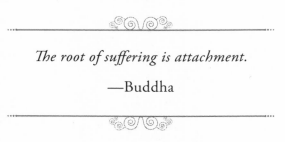

The root of suffering is attachment.

—Buddha

Attachment

1. a personal connection or feeling of kinship

2. the physical connection by which one thing is attached to another

3. a feeling of love or strong connection to someone or something

—Definitions sourced from 1) YourDictionary,
2) Merriam-Webster, and
3) Cambridge Dictionary.

In a Nutshell: Attachment is bonding or connecting with someone or something.

I f you sneak a peek inside my handbag, you will find I am still a lip-gloss girl and that I love the Clarins brand. You will also discover that I am a lady who likes quality pens and notebooks, has a bladder and bowel problem (I carry a 'Just Can't Wait' card from the Bladder and Bowel Community), and has a disability or health condition (I carry a medical alert card with information about my illness, the medication I take, and emergency contact details for my next of kin). Until you truly get to know me, chances are these things would label and shape the picture of the person you think I am.

While all these things are *part* of my life, none of them *are* me. And they are not the only labels that are or have been associated with my name. I have worn numerous descriptive labels throughout the years. Some have reflected my personality traits, my hobbies and interests, family roles, work, and job titles. In relation to health issues, the labels are varied, lengthy, and make for complex reading. Some labels have led me to withdraw into my shell, and at the other extreme, some have propelled me to take such bold action I have surprised myself.

You, too, have acquired specific labels. We all do.

Society uses labels every day to describe our ethnicity, religion, race, creed, colour, sex, and sexuality. Some labels identify health conditions or appearance, some come with job or family roles or titles, and others we consciously or inadvertently give ourselves.

We don't have to allow ourselves to be defined by the labels imposed on us. We get to define ourselves.

—Lizzie Velasquez

Your Labels May Be Different from Mine

Your labels may be quite different from mine; you may have different health conditions, physical challenges, or disabilities. People may see you as brave or frail, a born worrier, overweight or too thin. Maybe you are known as a health-food guru, a movie buff, an extrovert, or an introvert. The problem is not with the labels or titles themselves but with how we choose to interpret them and the burden any preconceived expectations, prognoses, or judgments these specific labels carry. It is all too easy to attach to our labels and start thinking, behaving, and acting in stereotypical ways.

Let me tell you about the day I was clinically diagnosed with multiple sclerosis (MS) and the impact that specific label had on my life.

It was a bleak autumn day in 1998, and I had received a phone message asking me to come in and see my general practitioner (GP) after his typical consulting hours to receive the results of some tests I'd had done a couple of weeks earlier. It was a wild and windy day, and I did not feel like going anywhere—but the health centre receptionist insisted.

When I arrived at the health centre, I sat alone in the empty waiting room for what seemed like a lifetime before I heard my doctor's footsteps approaching. Without directly looking at me, he called me by name and beckoned with a wave of his hand.

He was usually a chatty man, and I had always got on well with him. But that afternoon, he didn't speak as we made our way to his consulting room at the far end of the long narrowing corridor. The uneasy silence made me apprehensive of what was to come.

Once in his room, he invited me to take a seat, took a letter from his desk, and handed it to me. Then, saying he would come back in five minutes, he left me alone to read it. At the top of the letter, I saw my name and beside it in bold black type the words **Clinical Diagnosis Multiple Sclerosis.** Underneath there was a list of medications to be prescribed for me; 'these may be helpful as Maureen's symptoms progress.'

The letter said my recent MRI scan had been straightforward, but there had been neurological findings on my physical examination. Therefore, considering my 'prior and ongoing neurological medical history,' the specialist's opinion was that I had multiple sclerosis.

When my doctor returned, he asked me if my home had stairs. I told him it did, to which he responded, 'You'll need a bungalow with wide door frames. Most people with MS end up in a wheelchair within five years.'

He rummaged around in a drawer for a piece of paper. Finding one, he jotted down some figures and handed me the paper saying, 'If you need to get a house built or adapted, that's how wide the door frames need to be.'

I felt gutted, and at the same time, I felt a sense of déjà vu. Since I'd been told twelve years earlier that MS was a genuine possibility for me, the confirmation of the illness seemed inevitable. I had experienced debilitating fatigue and ongoing neurological symptoms for years after contracting a severe infection while on holiday in Mexico. My diagnosis was something I already felt prepared for and ready to handle. All the same, a massive wave of sadness washed over me as I thought of the life I was to lose.

My GP went on to tell me it was best I 'accept' my condition. There was no known cure for MS, and the most likely outcome would be that my illness would progress. I remember being asked several times if I understood the seriousness of his words and the impact on my future.

I said yes at the time (I guess it was what the doctor wanted to hear), and for the most part, I managed to keep my emotions together while in his consulting room. Ten minutes later, however, I could not help but notice how much heavier the health centre door felt as I left the building.

When I stepped outside, the cold air sliced through my body. I pulled my coat and scarf around me, desperately seeking comfort, and at a snail's pace, I painfully shuffled my way back to my car.

I was not thinking anything.

I was not doing.

A surreal numbness took over.

I struggled to find my car keys, and by the time I finally managed to get my car door open, I slumped into the driver's seat exhausted—as though someone had sucked the life out of me. Instinctively, I switched on the radio and turned it up to full volume, as if the music might stop me from having to think or feel.

It was late in the day, so there were no other cars or people around me. I sat there and sat there with the music playing loudly. I was not ready to go home or face the questions that would surely come from my family. I wondered whether this might all be a bad dream.

Eventually, I uncrumpled the scrap of paper my doctor had given me, still clutched in my hand. Through a blurry haze, I read the door frame measurements that would be required to facilitate wheelchair access. In that instant, my mental picture of my future changed. I saw a life of progressive weakness and disability—a life confined by a wheelchair and defined by pain.

Images appeared one by one in conjunction with the MS label I had been given: I saw myself as an old lady living in a bungalow relying on carers to bathe and dress me. I saw myself hobbling around on a stick and Zimmer frame and a wheelchair in my hall. I saw my mother and family having to look after me. I saw my frailty, ill health, and weakness. The pictures were real—and they were lifelike. I felt I was already in them. That was the moment the tears broke free. I sat alone in my car and cried for the future that lay ahead, for my family, and for the life I had not lived.

Fast forward a couple of years from that day, and I was precisely where I had predicted. I was registered 'disabled' and living in a bungalow with wide, wheelchair-access doorframes. The government had awarded me disability benefits for life as doctors did not expect my health to improve. I had a Motability car and a disabled parking badge.

I used a wheelchair to get around and relied heavily on carers. I spent most of my days within the four walls of my front room spaced out on a concoction of potent muscle relaxants and opioid drugs. Toileting issues had resulted in bowel surgery and a permanent stoma. Nurses had taught me how to catheterise my bladder and irrigate my bowels.

All conversations seemed to revolve around my illness. Friends and colleagues had disappeared from my life. I rarely saw anyone apart from my close family, carers, and medical professionals. It is amazing how quickly others started referring to me in conversation as 'Maureen, the lady with MS.'

That MS label stayed strongly attached to my name for the next fifteen years or so. And yet, today my doctors no longer use it. Medical opinions have evolved over time, and the MS label (previously seen as valid and applicable to me) has been unpeeled and replaced by several alternative health condition diagnoses. These diagnoses include degenerative disc disease and arthritis, bi-lateral neurogenic thoracic outlet syndrome, and an incurable systemic neurological condition—multi-site multi-system complex regional pain syndrome (CRPS). This severe central, peripheral, sympathetic, and autonomic nervous system dysfunction has been dubbed the 'suicide disease' because of its intense and excruciating pain levels (rated as the most severe known level of pain on the McGill Pain Index[5]).

DECIDE WHO YOU ARE

For all the labels I have worn through the years, I have learned that I can choose what identifiers I want to accept or own. I believe that you and I become what we are by being *who we are*—not the person others think we are or expect us to be.

The great composer Beethoven wrote beautiful music despite being labelled *deaf*. A divine spark of magic and genius resides in each of us. Only when we remove the unnecessary weight of our associated labels can we release our magic to the world.

Statements beginning with the words *I am* or *I have* are some of the most powerful statements you can say to yourself, especially when you attach yourself to the identifying words or phrases that follow. Phrases such as *I am disabled* or *I have a debilitating health condition* can put undue pressure on you to feel you have to behave, communicate, or live in expected ways.

You and I are so much more than any health condition or diagnosis anyone could ever give us. The problem is the stories we tell ourselves concerning our illness shape and colour the world in which we live.

You are not the labels that either you or others have given to you. Whether you unnecessarily restrict your world or commit to do all you can to expand your world does not come down to any descriptive label that may be associated with you.

Keeping Things Simple: The colour and size of your world and how fully you choose to live your life within it are shaped, steered, and defined by you.

RISE: SHED YOUR LABELS

*I am not my hair. I am not this skin. I
am the soul that lives within.*

—India.Arie, "I Am Not My Hair"

It is Day 2 of your elixir and time for your next assignment. Below, list any labels (health or otherwise) that are currently associated with you and that you believe hinder the life you live.

. . . .
. . . .
. . . .
. . . .
. . . .
. . . .
. . . .
. . . .

Once your list is complete, consider each label in turn and imagine peeling it away from the *true essence of you*. As you do so, imagine throwing each label away.

When you are done, breathe in some fresh energy and imagine dropping down deep within your body to reconnect with your soul, free of judgment and all labels. Finally, spend the next few minutes enjoying the newfound sense of freedom.

When you are ready, join me for Day 3.

DAY 3
REDIRECT YOUR THOUGHTS

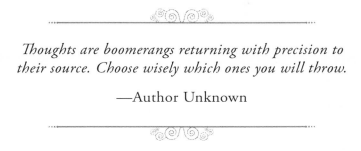

Thoughts are boomerangs returning with precision to their source. Choose wisely which ones you will throw.

—Author Unknown

Thought

1. an idea or opinion produced by thinking, or occurring suddenly in the mind

2. aim-oriented flow of ideas and associations that can lead to a reality-orientated conclusion

3. a form of energy and living data that is a facet of human consciousness which can have a specific cause and effect

> —Definitions sourced from 1) Lexico Dictionaries,
> 2) Wikipedia[6], and
> 3) Definitions.net.

In a Nutshell: Thought is the action and process of thinking, which allows you to make sense of or interpret the world you experience and make predictions about that world.

F acing your current reality and shedding restricting labels has brought you to a fantastic fresh starting place. From here on in, you have two main choices: feed the darkness or nurture and nourish the light.

Often, we can stay stuck in our circumstances simply because we get our thinking wrong. When we say, 'I am disabled. I suffer from fatigue. I am in pain and struggling,' the only thoughts and feelings we are likely to muster will focus on being disabled, suffering fatigue, and struggling with pain. In other words, without changing our thoughts, our feelings will remain the same.

With thoughts fixated on your illness or disability, you will find it difficult to open your mind to the possibility that you can have something different or better—better overall health, better quality of life, more heartfelt joy, more passion, more purpose, deeper contentment, greater strength and courage, more feelings of living fully alive and well.

> IF YOU ARE FEELING LOST, TRAPPED, OR STUCK IN LIFE, YOU ARE LIKELY TO STAY THERE IF YOU DO NOT REDIRECT YOUR THINKING.

The bottom line is this: if you are feeling lost, trapped, or stuck in life, you are likely to stay there if you do not *redirect your thinking*. Otherwise, all you will generate is more of the same old, same old if you do not open your mind to potentially having and feeling something else.

To fully embrace life, you must come alive to the possibility that the perceived limitations, predicted progress of symptoms, or expected prognosis of your specific illness or health condition may not be set in stone or 100 percent accurate. There is *always* something you can do to improve the overall quality of your well-being and health. That 'thing,' however, may only become apparent when you steer your thinking away from focusing on your illness or the problem itself and consciously redirect your thoughts to discovering, exploring, and taking the next best steps.

> *With everything that has happened to you, you can either feel sorry for yourself or treat what happened as a gift. Everything is either an opportunity to grow or an obstacle to keep you from growing. You get to choose.*

—Wayne Dyer

SMALL TWEAKS CAN REAP RICH REWARDS

Making small tweaks to your way of thinking is not challenging to do, and the impact of your new thoughts on the quality of your life can be enormous. Rather than overcomplicate things or put undue pressure on yourself, make simple changes slowly and one at a time. Living in pain is exhausting in itself; it can leave you feeling weak and your soul depleted. Rotten hours, days, or weeks happen. Sometimes there is no escaping bad days. That is *real life.*

We are only on Day 3, and I urge you to be kind to yourself by putting no pressure on yourself and keeping things doable. No matter your health condition or the daily challenges you face, choose to let some of the joy back into your life bit by bit—the playfulness and the peace and contentment your soul is craving. The key is to let go of the picture and story you have been telling yourself (of what you thought your life could or should be like or what you expect it may be in the future) and learn to create joy in your life that is *here, real,* and *now.* Wasting your valuable mental power on negative or unhelpful thoughts only blocks the light from streaming in.

E + R = O

I often share with my coaching and mentoring clients the equation *Event plus Response equals Outcome.* Unfortunately, the Event part of the equation is usually set in stone and something that we cannot go back and change. *Our response to that event remains flexible.* We can choose to think about or see an event differently; we can change our attitude, perception, and response. Although living with chronic pain and illness brings many challenges, changing your perception or thoughts about your experience will change how you feel and impact your actions, your quality of life, and the outcome you'll get.

BE WILLING TO START SOMEWHERE

You *deserve* to be happy—and if you are serious about experiencing more happiness in your life, you must commit to make positive changes and start somewhere! So choose today to laugh more than you cry, to love more than you hate, and to be grateful for what you can do rather than groaning about what you cannot do. Choose not to dwell in the darkness as the angry or bitter fighter but to evolve as the wise, courageous, graceful warrior. *Whether you choose to sing in life or complain about life, that choice always comes down to you.*

Keeping Things Simple: A brighter future is only ever a better quality of thought away.

RISE: REDIRECT YOUR THOUGHTS

You have power over your mind—not outside events. Realise this, and you will find strength.

—Marcus Aurelius

Minor changes to your way of thinking can significantly impact the quality of your life. Your Day 3 *Rise* assignment is simple: start becoming more aware of what you think and say. If a thought no longer serves you well or fails to bring you feel-good feelings, interrupt it, thank that thought for coming to your attention, tell it you no longer need it, and consciously choose to redirect your thoughts elsewhere.

PART TWO

AWAKEN

*Where do we even start on the daily walk
of restoration and awakening?*

We start where we are.

—Anne Lamott

DAY 4
HONOUR LIFE'S IMPERMANENCE

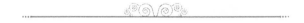

Life's impermanence, I realized, is what makes every single day so precious. It's what shapes our time here. It's what makes it so important that not a single moment be wasted.

—Wes Moore

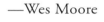

Impermanence

1. lack of permanence or continued duration

2. not permanent or enduring; transitory

3. the state or fact of lasting for only a limited period of time

> —Definitions sourced from 1) Wiktionary,
> 2) Dictionary.com, and
> 3) Lexico Dictionaries.

In a Nutshell: Impermanence is the state of not lasting forever or not lasting for a long time.

A breath comes, and in a second it is gone. A sensation—a burning or stabbing pain—arises and then quickly passes. A thought occurs, only to be replaced by another. Even the things we try convincing ourselves are here to stay and permanent are constantly changing, including our family and relationships, possessions, lifestyle, and experiences.

We are constantly changing. A Buddhist principle notes that everything changes. This reality is one of the few constants of which we can be certain. We are not always in control of what happens to us in life, whether we are born with a disability, get ill, become involved in an accident, or lose our job. Neither do we have control over the date we are born or the date of our death.

The world is a testament to impermanence
and uncertain futures; enjoy this day.

—Devin Waugh

The Tomorrows We Envision Do Not Always Get the Chance to Come

My father, Bruce, was only fifty-nine years old when he died. That's younger than I am now. He had planned to retire when he reached his sixtieth birthday but passed away before reaching that milestone—only a few months after receiving a cancer diagnosis.

His death was a shock to our family. His suffering, which seemed so cruel and pointless, awoke me to life's harsh reality. His last words to me were that life was precious and I must make the most of every day. He told me to enjoy life *now*, for tomorrow does not always get the opportunity to come.

> ENJOY LIFE NOW, FOR TOMORROW DOES NOT ALWAYS GET THE OPPORTUNITY TO COME.

I took his words to heart, knowing they were important, but grief and my personal health challenges stopped me from fully honouring them. The encouragement in those final words, however, never left me. They have helped me shape my life and make many lifestyle changes through the years. Indeed, they were the catalyst to me leaving an unhappy marriage and, after a few years on my own, meeting my amazing, soul-mate husband, Peter. My father's words instilled in me a deep desire to find happiness in my life *now* rather than waiting to find it somewhere down the line or allowing it to be dependent on better health or any future event.

In 2019, Peter was diagnosed with the same type of bowel cancer that took my father's life. Although externally I handled things very calmly, the first couple of weeks after Peter's diagnosis went by in a blur. When we first got the diagnosis, I had no idea whether I would have three more weeks, three more months, or three more years to be with the man I adored.

The ever-changing nature of life gave Peter and me profound level of appreciation for everything we held dear: the people we share life with, our beautiful home, the fantastic Scottish countryside we live in, the experiences our life had already brought us—and those it had yet to bring.

Within the space of love, we have voiced difficult conversations about life and death—conversations that have brought us an even deeper understanding of each other. As a result, we have awakened our perspective on life's meaning and value. To us, every single day feels like a truly precious gift.

We feel blessed that Peter's cancer was caught early and are so grateful for the skills and care of his excellent surgeon. Now, three surgeries later, I am delighted to tell you that Peter is cancer clear. And, God willing, we still have many more years to enjoy our lives together—and we are not going to waste a moment.

MAKE THE MOST OF EACH MOMENT

Fully understanding the impermanence of life brings home the beauty and preciousness of each moment. When you open your mind, eyes, and heart to the fact that you are never promised the tomorrow you envision, you do not want to waste a single day; you grow a burning desire to make each day count.

Any continuing difficult circumstances, pain, or health challenges you have diminish in their level of importance. As your soul whispers its reminder to *fully live* despite any challenge, you learn to passionately love and live more.

STANDING-ROOM ONLY—A FUNERAL FOR A FULL LIFE

Every pew in the church was filled on the day of my father's funeral. Every person I chatted with after the service spoke openly and warmly about my father and with love, respect, and kindness. No one mentioned his physical achievements or possessions; they talked about the type of person he was, what he gave to others, how true he was to himself, and what he gave to life.

Friends, family members, and colleagues poured out so much love for my father that day. I learned so much about him as they shared their memories. I had always known he was a wonderful father, doting grandfather, and loving husband to my mother. But on the day of his funeral, it became apparent to me he was also so much more.

Buddhists believe that people taken from this life at an early age are precious messengers sent to teach us about life's impermanence. As such, we are privileged to have known them and to have been part of their mission on earth.

Keeping Things Simple: Impermanence is the way of the Universe: things change all the time.

RISE: HONOUR LIFE'S IMPERMANENCE

When you truly embrace your human impermanence,
you connect with the power you have, and
influence you have, over the time you have.

—Steve Maraboli

Today's assignment is to project yourself forward in your mind towards the end of your life and imagine witnessing your funeral. What would you want to hear your family, loved ones, and friends say about you?

. . . .
. . . .
. . . .
. . . .
. . . .
. . . .
. . . .
. . . .
. . . .
. . . .
. . . .
. . . .
. . . .
. . . .
. . . .

DAY 5
GROW STRENGTH AND MENTAL RESILIENCE

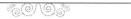

Anyone can give up; it's the easiest thing in the world to do. But to hold it together when everyone would expect you to fall apart, now that is true strength.

—Chris Bradford

Strength

1. the ability to do things that need a lot of physical or mental effort

2. the quality of being brave or determined in dealing with difficult or unpleasant situations

3. the capacity of an object or substance to withstand great force or pressure

> —Definitions sourced from 1) Cambridge Dictionary,
> 2) Longman Dictionary of Contemporary English Online, and
> 3) Lexico Dictionaries.

In a Nutshell: Strength is the quality or degree of being brave in difficult situations and being strong.

Last night was the night from hell. My feet and hands felt like they were in scorching lava, all four limbs were filled with stinging wasps and ants' nests. My head whooshed and pounded so rhythmically and dramatically that I feared it was going to explode. The intensity of the relentless, horrific pain made me feel certain I was burning alive from within. Every organ and limb felt on fire.

In desperation, I tried everything—from meditating and attempting self-hypnosis to putting on damp, cool flannels to using distraction techniques to repetitively uttering positive mantras. I don't normally swear, but last night, the words that involuntarily came out of my mouth were guttural and desperate.

Lying still beside my poor husband was nearly impossible. As excruciating muscle spasms increased their pace and frenzy, I went from sitting propped up by pillows and cushions— frightened to move for fear of further heightening the night's drama—to rocking back and forth, stark naked, desperately trying to dampen the raging bonfire in my nerves and bones on the cold tiles of the bathroom floor.

Sadly, my pain won last night. The hours were long and brutal. *The great thing, however, is that I got through them.* I made it through the eye of the storm and survived it. I am now in a new moment of a new day as I sit and write this morning. And for that, I am grateful and give thanks.

There is no doubt, however, the horrendous events of the night have taken their toll on me. I cannot deny that I have been depleted of desire *for anything* at this moment—I feel bruised and broken. I am not yet showered or dressed. My body feels too heavy, my brain too foggy, my soul dampened, my spirit struggling—my pain levels are still sky-high. The thought of carrying out the simplest of day-to-day tasks seems way too overwhelming. Last night's dark events severely tested my physical and mental resilience.

But, I am breathing. I am alive.

And dawn brings with it fresh light and hope by simply being here.

And I have come to realise that hope is precious.

However long the night, the dawn will break.

—African Proverb, Hausa Tribe

ALL MOMENTS PASS

In the depths of despair, when your pain is so severe it has you dropping to your knees begging for mercy, remind yourself that it won't last forever. The moment you are in is like all moments in life: it will pass.

I encourage you to accept that in those moments of crisis *it is as it is* for you. You are where you are, but you can and will get through it. Breathe from where you are and act from where you are. Remind yourself that you have endured acute pain before and survived it—and so you can survive it again today. When the voice in your head tells you that you cannot do this anymore, let hope and courage remind you, 'Yes, you can.'

> WHEN THE VOICE IN YOUR HEAD TELLS YOU THAT YOU CANNOT DO THIS ANYMORE, LET HOPE AND COURAGE REMIND YOU, 'YES, YOU CAN.'

What you tell yourself in these moments is hugely important, especially in the throes and aftermath of meltdown mayhem. The words, pictures, and thoughts you feed your brain have the power to lift you from where you are—to strengthen and comfort you—or to tear you down and lead you to doubt whether you can carry on. *In the world of chronic pain, the latter is not a helpful path to go down.*

You must believe in the possibility that you can and will get better and tell yourself that whatever life throws at you, you are strong enough to handle it. You must honour and respect the magic of your body—its ability to heal a cut all on its own, make your hair grow, and keep your heart beating without any effort from you.

Being strong is not about never feeling or experiencing pain. The strongest people are often those who feel their pain, fully understand it, and accept it whilst still enthusiastically committing to living their best life.

We *need* the bad times to direct us to look within ourselves. Experiencing challenges allows us to evolve and grow both emotionally and spiritually. It is our pain that makes our moments of joy more vibrant.

You and I are compassionate warriors, each on our unique path. We are carriers of much grit, grace, courage, and wisdom because of the difficult experiences we are going through. And after even the darkest of nights, the dawn always rises. Our crisis moments, crisis hours, crisis days, or crisis weeks may test us, but at some point, the light always cracks in once more, even if only ever so slightly, and breaks the darkest of nights.

DEVELOP MENTAL STRENGTH, RESILIENCE, AND COURAGE

When our pain screams and rears its ugliest and fiercest head, we need to dig deep with compassion and love for ourselves and rise strongly to meet it. We need to give our bodies their absolute best chance of surviving the crisis but also give our spirits what they need to thrive and heal. Mental resilience is one of the most critical attributes to reach that goal. If you doubt you have that kind of strength, I hope these truths will embolden you to believe you do—and that you can grow even stronger:

> ➢ Strength and mental resilience come from consistency of thoughts, beliefs, and actions—not from great dramatic feats, one-off efforts, giant steps of faith, or leaping over bridges or chasms.

> ➢ Mental resilience comes from the *doing* of mental resilience. Strength comes from the *doing* of being strong. You must build them gently and consistently by picking yourself up when you fall, whispering 'try one more time' when you feel like giving up, and telling yourself there will be a better day tomorrow when you think you cannot go on.

> ➢ Strength and mental resilience come from a deep-rooted hope and desire for life, a hunger for living, and a belief in the preciousness of your unique existence.

➤ Mental resilience, courage, and strength develop
not only with practice but also with the belief in the
divine power and soul alive within you.

In reviewing these truths, you'll notice that developing
mental strength, resilience, and courage happens in the
moment. That means you don't have to worry about the future
or the what ifs of tomorrow. All you need to do is hang on
as best you can in the moment you are in. Know you will get
through it. Believe you have the strength to handle it. This
moment, like all moments, whether good or bad, will pass.
Here are some strategies to help you rest in *this* moment.

BREATHE AND ALLOW YOURSELF TO FEEL WHAT YOU FEEL

Instead of fighting your pain, resisting it, or being overpowered
by it, accept it as it is for you in the moment. Allow yourself
to feel your pain and move through it.

When your pain levels are so high you feel scared or
anxious, interrupt the short, shallow chest-breathing pattern
of stress. Instead, try inhaling two quick breaths through your
nose followed by one long exhale through your mouth. Repeat
this pattern of two sharp inhalations followed by one longer
exhalation two or three times over. Alternatively, try slowing
your breathing down, imagine dropping down into the safe
place deep within your body, and visualise connecting with a
calm peace and stillness within.

Breathe and recognise that you have survived. A difficult moment has passed, and you had the strength to handle it. In the same way, you will have the power and strength to get through the next one. Imagine breathing in that strength— and as you exhale, let go of any thoughts or tension that no longer serves you well.

CHOOSE NOT TO FOCUS ON THE PAIN

Rather than focusing on the pain in the moment, choose to reflect on the grit, grace, and wisdom you have manifested in your most difficult moments.

Whatever you may have come to lack at a physical level, know that you have the power within you to compensate with an increase in your light and spirit. And as you connect with that spirit and shine its light forth, the magic happens—*it encourages others to do the same.*

Keeping Things Simple: Holding it together and moving with and through your pain—now that is true strength.

Rise: Grow Strength and Mental Resilience

Believe in yourself and all that you are. Know that there is something inside of you that is greater than any obstacle.

— Christian D. Larson

Strength, courage, and mental resilience come from the actual *doing* of strength, courage, and mental resilience. There is no other way.

So if you felt a little stronger now, had a little more courage now, a little more mental resilience, a little more hope for a better tomorrow, *how would you be acting now?*

Take a moment to reflect on your answer.

Your Day 5 *Rise* assignment is to go now and act in that way.

DAY 6
ADJUST YOUR MINDSET

Mind is a flexible mirror; adjust it, to see a better world.

—Amit Ray

Adjust

1. to put in good working order; regulate; bring to a proper state or position

2. to bring to a more satisfactory state

3. to change something slightly in order to make it better, more accurate, or more effective

—Definitions sourced from 1) Dictionary.com, 2) Merriam-Webster, and 3) Macmillan Dictionary.

In a Nutshell: To adjust means to move something to a better serving or more effective place.

P eople often ask me how I appear so happy when I live with a serious progressive neurological illness and experience constant pain. Unfortunately, the general misconception around appearing bright and cheerful is that all *must* be perfect in your world and that all is well.

Displaying a positive outlook can lead people—including family, friends, colleagues, and doctors—to form all sorts of preconceptions and opinions. Some people will believe that your symptoms cannot be so bad after all and that when you talk about your illness you are exaggerating its severity.

Exhibiting happiness when you live with intractable pain can often work against you and hinder you from getting the level of help and support you both deserve and need. That is a harsh truth and a real-life problem, but it is important not to let others' reactions or perceptions mould you into playing the victim to your situation or illness. There is no need to conform to others' ideas about how your condition should look or feel.

What many people fail to grasp is that genuine happiness is something deeply felt on the *inside*. Your mindset does not have to be determined by your physical body. Nor must it be dependent on events, happenings, or circumstances of your past or present world.

Happiness is so much more than a mood or emotion you feel. It is not as simple as a choice you make or a way of daily living. Happiness comes down to adjusting your perspective and being willing to open your eyes, mind, heart, and soul a little wider to see your world through a new, improved lens.

Happiness is the outcome of making a series of decisions that resonate positively within you on a soul level. Happiness is born from a growing awareness of who you are and what your valued and unique place is in this world.

Happiness is not exclusively available to those who are physically fit and healthy. Being happy is possible for every one of us, independent of our circumstances and our ailments, in the life each of us is living right here, right now.

> HAPPINESS COMES DOWN TO ADJUSTING YOUR PERSPECTIVE AND BEING WILLING TO OPEN YOUR EYES, MIND, HEART, AND SOUL A LITTLE WIDER TO SEE YOUR WORLD THROUGH A NEW, IMPROVED LENS.

Sometimes, life is what it is. How much better to accept that reality and experience happiness anyway rather than try to convince yourself otherwise. Despite what many mindset coaches may try to tell you, you are not in control of all things!

Coming to terms with living with chronic pain takes mental and physical adjustment. Although at times you may feel angry, sad, bitter, or hard done by, know that those feelings are natural and okay! Whatever health challenges you have or how much your physical body may be restricted, your circumstances do not destine you to a life of doom, gloom, and darkness. Likewise, your physical health conditions do not need to rob you of a rewarding life worth enthusiastically living. I promise that when you open your mind, heart, and soul to happier thoughts and feelings, happiness often finds its divine way of entering in.

No medicine cures what happiness cannot.

—Gabriel García Márquez

Keeping Things Simple: When you think happier thoughts, you feel happier; when you dwell on pain and sadness, you feel more pain and sadness. If you want to feel better about who you are and your place in the world, it is up to you to consciously adjust what you think and see.

RISE: ADJUST YOUR MINDSET

Folks are usually about as happy as they
make up their minds to be.

—Abraham Lincoln

For today's assignment, grab a pen and paper (or open a note on your phone) and find a quiet spot where you can be uninterrupted for about ten minutes.

Now list all the things you know make you feel happy, tend to make you feel better in some way, and lift your mood. If you are mentally not in the best place just now and need a major mood shift, aim to make as comprehensive and as lengthy a list as you can. It is amazing how many feel-good activities or happy memories can come to mind when you keep on asking yourself, 'And what else?'

Here are a few examples:

- I feel happy when I am near the sea.

- I get so much joy from talking to friends and being with family.

- I love snuggling up with a book and a milky coffee.

- Sitting in my garden is my happy place.

Take your time with this exercise, even if at first it feels a bit scary or difficult. Maybe all thoughts of being happy feel like a distant memory of a previous lifetime in a far-off world.

Notice as you list the things you enjoy how your mood shifts for the better. Choose to hang around for a while in your positive and feel-good imagination. When you are finished writing your list, read it over, shut your eyes, and see yourself doing one of those feel-good activities now.

DAY 7
NURTURE HOPE

Hope is being able to see that there is light despite all of the darkness.

—Desmond Tutu

Hope

1. an optimistic state of mind that is based on an expectation of positive outcomes with respect to events and circumstances in one's life or the world at large

2. to cherish a desire with anticipation: to want something to happen or be true

3. the feeling that what is wanted can be had or that events will turn out for the best

—Definitions sourced from 1) Wikipedia[7],
2) Merriam-Webster, and
3) Dictionary.com.

In a Nutshell: Hope is an outreaching desire with the expectancy of good.

There is no doubt—being in pain is exhausting. It can squeeze joy and the hope of a better tomorrow right out of you. Living with relentless and persistent pain is hard on your body, mind, spirit, and soul. Some days it feels as though you're shackled to a weight that keeps you from experiencing life.

How do I know this?

Because I experience those feelings too.

When each new day arises, so does your cruel companion. Pain accompanies you everywhere; there is no escape.

It may well be that doctors have told you there is little hope of your health condition or illness significantly improving. Some days, the absolute best you can do for yourself is get through the day—simply keep living and breathing—in the hope that tomorrow will be better and one day you will feel alive once more.

Hope—that one short, powerful word we are often robbed of—one of the most precious things we can ever possess.

Hope is like the first flowers of spring and the scent of the most beautiful rose in your garden. Hope is the wonder in children's eyes when they discover something beautiful or magical for the first time. It is the shining star emerging from the darkest sky, the all-important component that can propel you onwards however challenging or painful your circumstances may be.

With hope, the magic of life still looks available to you. For with hope, fresh new opportunities and better times ahead remain possible.

Without hope, you risk being drained of all energy; many doors will appear bolted and impossible to open. Locked behind those doors, you risk settling for a life limited by negative expectations.

Your pain is real, as is my pain. There is no getting around that. There is no disputing that.

But hope is real also. And it is important to acknowledge that truth.

Hope is not about pretending your pain and illness do not exist or impact your life. It is about believing that things can improve for you. All hope asks of you is to make the most positive use you can of your present whilst optimistically remaining open to experiencing nourishing and rewarding times ahead.

Hope is not something for which you or I can go shopping. You cannot pick hope like a ripe apple from a heavily laden fruit tree. Neither is it something that anyone else can give to you if you are not in the right place mentally to receive it. Hope is something that ignites within. It is something you must consciously choose to nurture.

> HOPE IS SOMETHING THAT IGNITES WITHIN. IT IS SOMETHING YOU MUST CONSCIOUSLY CHOOSE TO NURTURE.

Once you choose hope, everything is possible.

—Christopher Reeve

You Lose Nothing by Nurturing Hope

Living with hope costs nothing and makes for a richer, fuller, enlivened life experience. Even if hope does not lead to the level of significant physical improvement you may long for, it will enable you to live optimistically and joyfully each precious day.

For that reason, I choose to keep the doorway of hope in my heart and mind open wide. The hope that fuels my spirit and soul also enables me to recognise the many blessings the Universe brings me.

Hope is precious. Even a single thread of hope is worth hanging on to. Guard your hope fiercely. Do not let others diminish your hope with their words or actions. *An optimistic mind is a vitalizing life force and an empowering thing.*

Keeping Things Simple: It is in the presence of hope that better times, magic, and miracles can enter. In hope's presence, the light streams in.

RISE: NURTURE HOPE

*When the world says, 'Give up,' Hope
whispers, 'Try it one more time.'*

—Author Unknown

Your Day 7 *Rise* assignment is to take a few minutes to rest
and reflect and explore what having more hope of a better
tomorrow could mean to you. Use the following statements
as prompts (simply fill in the blanks):

With more hope, I might be

. . . .

. . . .

. . . .

. . . .

. . . .

. . . .

With more hope, I might feel

. . . .

. . . .

. . . .

. . . .

. . . .

. . . .

With more hope, I might do

. . . .
. . . .
. . . .
. . . .
. . . .
. . . .

With more hope, the following might become a little easier or possible for me

. . . .
. . . .
. . . .
. . . .
. . . .
. . . .

Pull those thoughts into your present moment by shutting your eyes and crafting a mental image of yourself doing and feeling the things you have explored and imagined. See yourself moving positively forwards and emanating a hope renewed, nourished, and brightly burning.

DAY 8
LIVE IN YOUR NOW

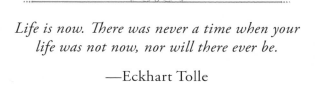

*Life is now. There was never a time when your
life was not now, nor will there ever be.*

—Eckhart Tolle

Now

1. at the present time, not in the past or future

2. of or relating to the present time

3. of the present or current time

—Definitions sourced from 1) Cambridge Dictionary,
2) Merriam-Webster, and
3) YourDictionary.

***In a Nutshell: Now is this exact moment, here and present,
that you and I are currently in.***

I t is all too easy to look back on your life with the 'I wish that had never happened . . . I wish I had never done that . . . what if this had happened instead' outlook.

It is natural to grieve for the life you used to live, the better health you enjoyed, the type of person you may have been then, and the level of independence and freedom you may previously have experienced.

The thing about the past is that it has passed—and there is nothing you or I can do now to go back and change things. We cannot rerun past events or erase significant happenings in our life. We can reframe how we think about them (and that can certainly help our souls and spirits healing from them), but we cannot change what has physically happened.

What happened has happened. What passed is now over. What may have happened to you in the weeks, months, or years gone by is now history—a time passed and gone.

THE FUTURE CAN BE SCARY

When shall we live, if not now?

—Seneca

Thoughts of what may happen in the future can be scary, especially when you are seeing through dark lenses of pain and illness. Your mind can manifest and multiply anxious thoughts and pictures of *what, when*, and *might be*. Your thoughts can run away with you if you do not take conscious ownership of them and choose to gently guide and steer them in a nurturing and beneficial direction. Your life is only ever as good as you allow your personal experience of it to be.

TIME—FACTS AND TRUTH

The past has passed—and it is over. The future is not here yet—it exists in your mind only. You cannot save up the time from a bad health or flare day to enjoy on a better health day. You cannot cut a couple of hours from a dark and gloomy day to stick at the end of another.

That is not the way life and time works.

Time itself exists (events happen and everything gets older), but in terms of years, months, days, hours, minutes, and seconds, time is a man-made construct. None of us gets preferential treatment. Whilst we are alive on this earth, we all have the same sixty minutes in an hour and twenty-four hours in a day to experience and live as best we can.

ONLY NOW IS TRUE AND REAL

It is only in the moments that arise *in your now* that you can breathe, eat, sleep, and nourish yourself; experience rewarding relationships; fully embrace who you are; evolve, learn, and grow; love and free your spirit; and make your next best choices.

If you want to look back on your life feeling you have given it your best shot, then the only time you can live that best life is in the moment currently unfolding before you. The moment that was here a minute ago is already gone. Each moment flows into memory as each new moment enters. When each moment is over, it can never be repeated in the same way, time, or space as before.

And that, my reader, is something quite magical when you get your head around it, for it means life presents us constantly with new opportunities. It is never too late for fresh new beginnings and new ways of thinking. At any point, we can choose to start doing things differently and become an even more awesome version of the person we were born to be.

> AT ANY POINT, WE CAN CHOOSE TO START DOING THINGS DIFFERENTLY AND BECOME AN EVEN MORE AWESOME VERSION OF THE PERSON WE WERE BORN TO BE.

In truth, most of us can put ourselves through more suffering in our minds and imagination than exists in our present-day reality. Viewing our life backwards or forwards through eyes of disappointment, regret, anxiety, or fear can mean we miss out on seeing the beauty, learning, or gift that the Universe is doing its best to present. We can miss out on appreciating the little things that bring us joy, noticing the gentle touch of love, hearing the whisper in our ear of our innermost desires and callings. We can fail to hear the birdsong in our garden or savour the wonderful scent of newly baked bread or fresh cut flowers.

LIFE IS A PARTICIPATORY EVENT

Making the most of life comes down to actively participating in life and the daily *doing* of more enlivened living. You and I may not have chosen the cruel companion of pain or illness, but whether we see our life as going *nowhere* because of it or seeing life as *now here* for us is a perception and choice only we can make.

Your mind is your mind. Your physical body is your body. It is your world that you live in, as I live in my world. If we want to live our best life, however, we must make *living* a mind–body–spirit–soul experience. We must throw ourselves fully and completely into life and consciously embrace it despite any difficulties it may present along the way. Retreating to the side-lines is not going to encourage the high levels of happiness and joy we deserve.

SOMETHING PRACTICAL YOU CAN DO TO HELP

If you have been struggling to embrace life as it is for you and fully live it, write down any significant past events or circumstances about which you have regrets or that you still feel bitter, hurt, angry, sad, or guilty about. Get any negative experiences that have happened in your life down on paper and *out of you.*

When you are finished with your list, write this boldly across it:

> I forgive myself completely and wholeheartedly for keeping alive any unhelpful or negative energy surrounding my past events and circumstances. What has happened in the past has passed and is over. I let go of what no longer serves me well.

Burn your list, rip it up ceremoniously, or bury it in the garden. Scream and shout if you want to or celebrate with a glass of wine or bubbly. Make letting go of negative thoughts around your past a significant and empowering occasion. Whatever happens naturally for you at this time, simply let it happen. When your gamut of emotions has run its course, consciously choose to sit quietly in mindful reflection and breathe in the feeling of renewed fresh mental space and energy. In the simple ceremonious act of letting your negative thoughts around your past go, your mood and mindset will lift and lighten, and a newfound enthusiasm for life will begin to emerge.

Keeping Things Simple: Life is not a movie playing out behind you, in front of you, or somewhere over there. Every single minute you spend dwelling in what was, what might have been, or your what might be is a precious minute less for you to embrace what is true and now here.

RISE: LIVE IN YOUR NOW

Nothing is but what is now.

—Ron Rash

Your Day 8 assignment is to slow your breathing and notice what is real in this present moment. Jot down your observations below.

Five things I see now:

1.

2.

3.

4.

5.

Five things I hear now:

1.

2.

3.

4.

5.

Five things I taste or smell:

   1.

   2.

   3.

   4.

   5.

Five things I am touching and can feel:

   1.

   2.

   3.

   4.

   5.

Now sit for a few moments keeping your focus fully in your present—experiencing, noticing, and feeling what is real and here for you.

Feel the floor or chair beneath you.

Feel the temperature of the air around you.

Feel your heart beating.

Feel your soul speaking.

Gently breathe a little more deeply and open your awareness even further—notice all that is here for you now and present.

DAY 9
LIVE IN THE BREATH

If you want to conquer the anxiety of life,
live in the moment, live in the breath.

—Amit Ray

Breath

1. the air that goes into and out of your lungs

2. spirit or vitality

3. the power of breathing; life

—Definitions sourced from 1) Cambridge Dictionary,
2) American Heritage Dictionary, and
3) Lexico Dictionaries.

In a Nutshell: Breath is an inhalation or exhalation of air from your lungs especially necessary to live.

When the future seems too terrifying to contemplate and the past is too painful to remember—I remind myself the only moment that requires my attention is this moment I am in, right here, right now.

I remind myself that I am safe; I am not alone. I awaken my senses and breathe in the fresh moment as it enters. I consciously align myself to see, hear, taste, touch, and feel what is real and now here.

Nothing else matters at this moment. As I realign myself with my present, I drop down from my over-thinking brain to connect with my soul and distance myself from my physical body. Within the safe sanctuary that lies within me, I notice how peaceful and calm I feel.

Any prior feelings of overwhelm gently start to leave me.

Any feelings of anxiety or tension disperse and float off into the distance.

In the times when my pain raises its fiercest fire, mindful moment-by-moment living and focusing on one breath at a time is proving a vital lifeline. It is all too easy otherwise for my pain to take over and instigate a mental cacophony of images of what may or may not come.

And so, I choose to breathe in these moments and feel what I feel.

I choose to acknowledge my pain for its presence only and let go of all judgment about whether it is fair or unfair, good or bad for me. Thus, I do not feel the need to number its severity on a pain scale from one to ten (as doctors and medical professionals often ask us to do). I focus on and live in the breath I am in right now, for I know this moment will soon be gone and replaced by the next new moment that enters.

In life—especially in the world of living with pain and illness—one moment, one breath, one next best step at a time, is all we ever need to do. It is not about fighting, denying, or blocking pain. It is about moving through pain—and moving with it—with focused breathing and a moment-by-moment awareness shifting all attention away from the core of our pain to our breath and a more soul-gratifying thought or action. It is about taking ownership of our pain and gently steering and guiding it towards a deeper, relaxed, more manageable, and comfortable place.

> ONE MOMENT, ONE BREATH, ONE NEXT BEST STEP AT A TIME, IS ALL WE EVER NEED TO DO.

Accessing that more comfortable place is not always easy. Sometimes we must learn to embrace and fully live our lives alongside pain's presence as an ever-demanding and challenging companion, tagging along with a firm grip on us.

With time, however, and with a lot of self-love, self-care, self-compassion, understanding, letting go, forgiveness, and inner emotional healing—blended seamlessly with a bank of practical and effective pain management strategies—pain and illness can be encouraged to take up less room in your life. Managing your pain better frees up space for more joy, peace, inspired passion, purpose, and laughter, with less fear and anxiety. As you recognise what matters, you also experience deeper contentment. Managing your pain better both frees and empowers you to live with more enthusiasm and develops greater confidence in your ability to handle whatever the future may bring.

Although my physical health has progressively deteriorated, I feel alive and *soul well*. Learning to access the safe, serene stillness within my breath has proved to be my lifeline. Ten minutes of sitting quietly and focusing on my breathing has become a non-negotiable part of my day.

> ALTHOUGH MY PHYSICAL HEALTH HAS PROGRESSIVELY DETERIORATED, I FEEL ALIVE AND SOUL WELL.

Whatever is currently going on in your life, consciously breathe into it—allow yourself to feel what you feel, letting go of all thought or judgement. Put loving arms around yourself. Slow your breathing, and as you do so, gently drop your shoulders. Now, breathe a little slower and deeper. Consciously shift your focus inwards and enjoy the feelings of calm and peace.

Another world is not only possible; she is on her way. On a quiet day, I can hear her breathing.

—Arundhati Roy

Keeping Things Simple: More ease and grace, more peace and comfort, are only ever a breath away.

RISE: LIVE IN THE BREATH

Sometimes the most important thing in a whole day
is the rest we take between two deep breaths.

—Etty Hillesum

Your Day 9 assignment is to follow this simple step-by-step breathing exercise, which will almost instantaneously help ease any feelings of anxiety, overwhelm, stress, or discomfort.

1. Gently breathe in through your nose for the count of two.

2. Hold the still space of the breath for the count of two.

3. Breathe out through your mouth for the count of five whilst saying in your mind the word *relax.*

Repeat the above three steps another two or three times (to a maximum of four repetitions if you feel a little lightheaded), developing awareness of how more deeply relaxed you are beginning to feel.

As you are able, gently stretch your limbs. With your next breath in, visualise the vitality of a fresh spring morning entering your body. Then, as you breathe out, imagine letting go of any remaining negative energy that no longer serves you well.

Rest for a moment and enjoy all that the power of breath has brought you. Notice how much more peaceful and comfortable you now feel.

If you would like to know more about using the power of consciously controlled breathing (often referred to as meditation), visit my website to download a free meditation audio: MaureenSharphouse.com.

DAY 10
LOOK INSIDE, BE PROUD

You really have to look inside yourself and find your own inner strength and say, 'I'm proud of what I am and who I am'.

—Mariah Carey

Proud

1. having, proceeding from, or showing a high opinion of one's own dignity, importance, or superiority

2. feeling happy about your achievements, your possessions, or people who you are connected with

3. having proper self-respect

—Definitions sourced from 1) Dictionary.com,
2) Macmillan Dictionary, and
3) Merriam-Webster.

In a Nutshell: Being proud means having a heartfelt feeling of your self-respect and personal worth.

When you feel that your physical body lets you down, it can be difficult to maintain self-esteem and pride in yourself. Facing each day with less energy and physical ability can eat away your confidence and deplete your enthusiasm for life. As a result, you may find yourself sitting on the side-lines feeling stuck and encased as if in a restrictive bubble. At the same time, the rest of the world seems to be moving forwards with their lives—your colleagues advance in their careers, and your friends and family members carry on enjoying everyday activities with ease.

As much as you try to convince yourself and others that you are happy, you find yourself yearning to feel normal again. Your former life takes on a rosy glow in your memory; you start longing for the seemingly more perfect past. When you see yourself as less worthy in some way, however, a vital part of your soul becomes dampened. As your enthusiasm and love for life wanes, fear, exhaustion, and self-defeating thoughts open you up to being soul depleted. If those thoughts continue, the hunger for life in your soul may well be extinguished as you lose a piece of what makes you *you*.

The problem is, the more you feel lost, the more your soul urges you to fill that void so you can feel alive again. It is all too easy to attempt to fill the void with material things and busyness, bingeing on daytime television or Netflix, overspending, or giving in to unhelpful addictions such as excessive use of cigarettes, alcohol, food, or drugs.

None of these things will rekindle your soul's fire. Whilst comfort eating, the use of recreational or prescription drugs, or downing a bottle of wine may numb the pain for a short time, no external remedy has the power to carry a more positive sense of the *real you* to your world.

> *If you are always trying to be 'normal' you will*
> *never know how amazing you can be.*

—Maya Angelou

THE SECRET

The secret to feeling good about yourself again is to learn to love yourself as you are. Pride in who and what you are and feeling soul well and happy only manifests when you are brave enough to be real with yourself.

PRIDE IN WHO AND WHAT YOU ARE AND FEELING SOUL WELL AND HAPPY ONLY MANIFESTS WHEN YOU ARE BRAVE ENOUGH TO BE REAL WITH YOURSELF.

THE GREATEST GIFT

The greatest gift you can ever give yourself is permission to be the person you are capable of being. Each one of us is perfectly imperfect in some way. Having a perfect body, enjoying excellent health, or living an ideal life is not the reality of our world. Perfect is not *real life.*

We each have our quirks, strengths, weaknesses, talents, skills, preferences, interests, passions, and abilities. No matter how oppressed by our pain and illness we may feel at times, there is no need to darken the colours of the world in which we live. It is up to each one of us to own our story, live and tell it well, and fulfil our unique place in the world. Each of us must stand in our reality and truth rather than shy away from or deny it. No matter the extent of your challenges, you are the only one who can relegate yourself to the back seat of life. You still have a legacy to live and a story to tell. There is no requirement to become the disillusioned spectator of others who are seemingly having greater success or fun.

YOU ARE A UNIQUE CREATION

You are a unique creation and a gift from God. Your physical body is only the suit you wear—the channel through which your soul operates. You are beautiful. You are amazing. You are a divine gift to the world and are whole and perfect. You are enough as you are, for you are a beacon of true courage, grit, grace, and strength.

Keeping Things Simple: Whilst your current physical health condition may impact your body's ability to do certain things or affect your external appearance in some way, your unique strength, spirit, and soul remain secure deep within you. There will only ever be one of you; no one can do you for you. It is up to you to look inside and say, 'I am proud of who and what I am.'

RISE: LOOK INSIDE, BE PROUD

Take pride in yourself. Be your own person.

—Jack Lambert

For your Day 10 assignment, get comfortable in your favourite chair. Below, list ten things you are proud of yourself for—both the small and the large.

I am proud of myself for these things:

1 . . . .
 . . . .

2 . . . .
 . . . .

3 . . . .
 . . . .

4 . . . .
 . . . .

5 . . . .
 . . . .

6 . . . .
 . . . .

7 . . . .
 . . . .

8 . . . .
. . . .

9 . . . .
. . . .

10 . . . .
. . . .

Once you have finished the list, please take a moment to read it through. Then reflect on what you have achieved so far in life and what you achieve daily. Pat yourself on the back. You deserve it!

Give some thought to what you can do as you move forward to be even prouder of yourself being *you*.

PART THREE

RESTOKE

*The secret to change is to focus all your energy not
on fighting the old but on building the new.*

—Socrates

DAY 11
REIGNITE YOUR PASSION

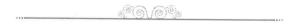

*There is no passion to be found playing small—in settling
for a life that is less than the one you are capable of living.*

—Nelson Mandela

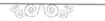

Passion

1. a strong or extravagant fondness, enthusiasm, or
   desire for anything

2. something that produces a strong enthusiasm or
   interest in you

3. intense, driving, or overmastering feeling or
   conviction

—Definitions sourced from 1) Dictionary.com,
2) Macmillan Dictionary, and
3) Merriam-Webster.

**In a Nutshell: Passion is an emotion and feeling fuelled by
doing what you have a strong desire or interest in and enjoy.**

If you are currently struggling to break free from the dark shadows of pain and illness, doing more of the things that matter to you and fire the feeling of joy and passion can be a real game-changer. It can change how you feel about yourself and the quality of your daily life.

Without passion, you are likely to have more and more 'bad days' when you do not feel like getting out of bed, cannot be bothered to get dressed, put off showering, and fail to feed yourself well. As a result, you are more likely to start living like a hermit, avoiding friends and relationships, experience mental anxiety, or find yourself feeling let down by life and become suicidal or depressed.

While your pain and illness may have altered or significantly changed your life, this does not mean your enthusiasm for living a life with passion must also change. What matters to you matters! Following your heart and doing more of the things that bring you joy will not only positively impact your overall health and well-being—it will bring a sense of purpose and a deeply rooted fulfilment to your day.

Passion is the bridge that takes you from pain to change.

—Frida Kahlo

PASSION IS YOUR HEALING MEDICINE

Passion is not something that can be found by thinking about it in your head; you must make it a full mind/body/spirit/ soul experience and *do* what stirs the feel-good feelings in you. Passion is the medicine that can take you from hurt to healing and the catalyst for you to feel enthusiastic about life again rather than simply existing or going through the daily motions of getting by.

THE MOST BEAUTIFUL PEOPLE ARE SOULS ALIVE

If you find yourself somewhat apprehensive of what I say, it is worth reminding yourself that the most beautiful people in the world are not the ones with seemingly perfect bodies or preened external appearance. Neither are they those with the greatest physical or mental ability or with the highest IQ. The most beautiful people in the world are those who emanate a charisma or presence—they are the souls visibly alive, the human souls on fire with a glimmering sparkle in their eyes.

PASSION HAS POWER

Whilst you may have to do things a little differently than before, you will find many activities that you *can do* that have the power to bring about positive and empowering feelings. The physical experience of doing more of the things that stir desire and joy in you will lead you on the path to feeling alive again and soul well.

Here is a list of the things that are important to me and make my life feel fulfilling and rewarding:

- writing and journaling

- cooking and baking

- knitting

- playing the piano

- listening to music (loudly!)

- being out in nature

- fresh flowers

- the sound of birdsong

- the beauty of sunrises and sunsets

- the beautiful animals I share my life with

- valuable friendships

- the time I spend with my husband and family

Call these my passions; call them my joys. Whatever you choose to call them is not what is important. What is important is that you do things (either on your own or with others) that speak to your heart, feel good to you, excite or inspire you, light the spark of fire within you, and naturally feel like home.

START FROM WHERE YOU ARE

If you have been ill for some time, feelings of passion may seem quite alien to you. That is okay—start from where you are. Reconnect with old things and keep trying new ones. If some activities you used to love to do in life are no longer easy or possible for you, do not let that detract or distract you—*surf possibilities.* It does not need to be big or something that others perceive as important. It does not need to be something that appealed to you when you were more physically able or much younger.

PASSIONS ARE NOT FIXED

Passions and interests in life are not fixed. They are fluid and flexible—they grow and change with us as we mature and get older and as our circumstances and situations change.

What are the things that catch your heart? What speaks to your soul? Who and what brings a smile to your face and stirs feel-good feelings?

If you want to feel better about yourself and reignite the fire of passion within you, you must do more things that bring that warmth and light into your life.

YOU CAN CLUCK, OR YOU CAN FLY

If you hang out with chickens, you're going to cluck and if you hang out with eagles you're going to fly.

—Steve Maraboli

When you start to participate more in activities to fire your passion and enthusiasm for life, it is important to surround yourself with people who inspire, encourage, and support you—the ones who feel like sunlight. You will not find it beneficial to mix with those who demotivate, fatigue, drain you, fail to add something positive to your experience, or pull you down.

Let us get clear: You are allowed to have fun; you are allowed to be creative. You are allowed to laugh; you are allowed to have a passion for life.

Whilst you may have a chronic health condition and some activities may not come so easily for you, spending time with others who do not

> DOING MORE OF THE THINGS THAT STIR DESIRE AND JOY IN YOU WILL LEAD YOU ON THE PATH TO FEELING ALIVE AGAIN AND SOUL WELL.

wholly support your desire to create more joy in your life will not help your overall well-being. Nor will they beneficially nourish your mind, body, spirit, heart, and soul.

Keeping Things Simple: Your strength lies within your passion. Do not let pain and illness restrain you from spilling forth to the world all that you are.

RISE: REIGNITE YOUR PASSION

The most powerful weapon on earth is the human soul on fire.

—Ferdinand Foch

It is Day 11, and your *Rise* assignment today is to jot down below the creative activities that have the power to uplift your mood and spirits. Think about what you used to love to do and enjoy—and explore the possibilities of what may be feasible to recommence (or alternatives that would bring you similar feel-good feelings).

. . . .

. . . .

. . . .

. . . .

. . . .

. . . .

. . . .

. . . .

. . . .

. . . .

. . . .

Now surf new interests or activities that excite or appeal to you that perhaps you have never had the time or opportunity before to try. Be brave and bold. Do not let your current health hold you back. Write them down!

. . . .

. . . .

. . . .

. . . .

. . . .

. . . .

. . . .

. . . .

. . . .

. . . .

Once you have captured your thoughts, shut your eyes and see yourself in your mind actively enjoying and doing one of those things now.

DAY 12
EMBRACE ALIVE

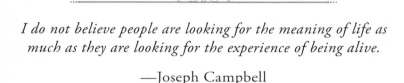

I do not believe people are looking for the meaning of life as much as they are looking for the experience of being alive.

—Joseph Campbell

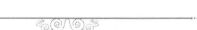

Alive

1. living and not dead : still existing and not gone or forgotten

2. having life : not dead or inanimate

3. possessing life, full of spirit

—Definitions sourced from 1) YourDictionary, 2) Merriam-Webster, and 3) Princeton's WordNet.

In a Nutshell: The state of being physically alive means not being dead.

When my father died some thirty years ago, I felt
I had to be strong for my mother and family.
I blocked and resisted the emotions wrestling
within me; I feared feeling their full intensity would cause
me to crumble and collapse with the pain. I did all I could to
keep on living, to get by each day, to go through the motions.
But, in truth, I became numb. I was one of the living dead.
I was doing no more than acting on automatic pilot: getting
up, getting dressed, seeing my children off to school, going
to work, coming home, making dinner, tidying up, sitting in
front of the television, taking no joy or interest in what I was
watching or doing, washing, undressing, and each evening
tumbling exhausted into bed.

I watched my mother regularly fall to her knees, not
wanting to face another day or open her bedroom curtains. I
was frightened of experiencing that depth of grief myself—
terrified of falling into the same dark cavern of the inconsolable
sadness it was evident she felt. It wasn't until several years later
that I broke down uncontrollably and let my tears flow freely.
The release of those tears and fully feeling the raw pain of my
own emotions sparked my heart to begin to heal.

I started to wake up as if from a long sleep; I noticed how
much my son had grown and how much my daughter's hair
glistened. Then, bit by bit, I began to smile again, feel alive
again, laugh again, and openly cry again.

During the years from my father's death up to that point,
I was not fully living. I was doing what I needed to do to

get through each day—but my soul and spirit felt dull and depleted.

The problem was I had been blocking out reality and shielding myself from the pain that was true and real to me. I was trying to hide from my own emotions by falsely putting on a brave and happy face to the world.

Inside, there was no calm or peace for me, no grace and gratitude, no passion or enthusiasm for life. All that grew within me were niggling doubts about faith and a feeling of being let down by the Universe and God.

Death and grief are natural parts of life and elements of the human experience. Being fully alive means being alive to *all* life's moments—not only the ones you like or prefer or choose for yourself.

Humans are sensual beings, experiencing the world we live in by sensing and feeling. Living alive requires more than breathing, going through the daily motions, and enjoying the odd passionate moment. It is more than having enjoyable evenings with friends, knowing we have a lot to be grateful for, or experiencing a better day. A heart beating and lungs breathing are never enough on their own. Being fully alive requires participating in life completely—you must involve yourself in life with your whole self.

> BEING FULLY ALIVE REQUIRES PARTICIPATING IN LIFE COMPLETELY—YOU MUST INVOLVE YOURSELF IN LIFE WITH YOUR WHOLE SELF.

Living alive comes not only from creating joy and meaning in your life but also from your willingness to embrace the good moments and the sad, bad, or painful ones. It comes from embracing the exciting, inspiring, and happy moments as well as the difficult, boring, and mundane.

To *feel* alive, you must *do* and *be* alive. There is no other way. You must actively participate no matter what joy or pain life may bring you. You must allow yourself to fully experience the true emotions you feel and not shun or hide away from them in denial or fear.

Being alive can feel joyous; it can also be hurtful.

Being alive may feel sad at times and somewhat painful.

To *feel,* however, is one of our greatest gifts. Breathing life into your soul comes from experiencing all that life offers, including its intensity and unpredictability. To be alive to life, you must learn to ride the waves. You must walk through life's storms and trust the darkness. You must take things as they come and allow yourself to enter these moments with a heart open to feel them.

There is no need to turn life into drama. The magic that makes the difference is accepting and embracing the reality of what is going on while respecting and honouring your personal feelings, vulnerability, and truth.

Keeping Things Simple: Feeling alive is the reward that manifests from wholeheartedly embracing the full range and depth of emotions that as souls on earth we have been gifted with.

RISE: EMBRACE ALIVE

*What makes you feel alive is your truth. What
makes you come alive is your truth.*

—Oprah Winfrey

Your assignment for Day 12 is to ask yourself the following
questions and jot down your answers below. There is no need to
show anyone what you have written. Use this as your safe place
to explore your innermost emotions, feelings, and thoughts.

Questions to Self

**How soul awake and alive am I? (Circle your answer on a
scale of 1 to 10 with 10 being the highest.)**

1   2   3   4   5   6   7   8   9   10

**In what aspects of life am I simply existing and going
through the motions day by day?**

. . . .
. . . .
. . . .
. . . .
. . . .
. . . .

What am I hiding from, protecting myself from, blocking, fearing, avoiding, or resisting?

. . . .
. . . .
. . . .
. . . .
. . . .
. . . .

What is it that I need to allow myself to experience more fully, accept the truth of, or do?

. . . .
. . . .
. . . .
. . . .
. . . .
. . . .

If your answers leave you feeling a little uncomfortable, know that the time will come when you start to feel alive again. In the meantime, simply keep on living one day at a time. Consciously get more involved with life. Be kind and patient. Living fully alive is not solely dependent on your heart beating but on your soul's willingness to fully embrace everything life brings.

DAY 13
VALUE YOUR BIRTHRIGHT

The privilege of a lifetime is to become who you truly are.

—Carl Jung

Privilege

1. a right or immunity granted as a peculiar benefit, advantage, or favor

2. an opportunity to do something special or enjoyable

3. something regarded as a special honour

> —Definitions sourced from 1) Merriam-Webster,
> 2) Cambridge Dictionary, and
> 3) Lexico Dictionaries.

In a Nutshell: Freedom to be who you truly are is a right and privilege to which you are entitled by birth.

As I write these words, I am sitting in my garden writing, listening to the wind rustle through the leaves on the trees. The words of a Jewish proverb come to mind: 'Every blade of grass has its angel that bends over it and whispers, "Grow, grow."' I hear a soft, internal whisper, 'Maureen, *grow.*'

Growth marks life's journey. As we meet challenges, they stretch us. Some experiences we encounter on our path awaken our senses, stir our emotions, shape our feelings, and influence our thoughts. Life events can also be hurtful and upsetting. In the moment, it can be hard to see the blessings from those painful situations. Those times, however, provide us with wisdom and the strength to grow.

As I look back on my life, I can see a journey of highs and lows. Although I may not always have recognised the learning in the moment, with hindsight, I can see how my experiences and the knowledge I have gained from them have brought me to a place of ever-deepening awareness of a bigger presence all around me and the appreciation of the soul and spirit within me. With that awareness, a soothing peace lies within me, comforting me even on the most difficult days.

YOU HAVE A CHOICE NOW. WE ALL DO.

You have a choice in life to expand or contract. You can embrace the lessons and gifts offered to you in life, or you can inadvertently contain your world and remain blind to them. You can become more of who you are meant to be and be more of who you truly are—or you can crawl into your shell, stay stuck down a dark hole, live overshadowed by darkness, or at best live in shades of grey.

As I have been writing these words, the sun has been shining. Dark clouds have made fleeting visits, however, as I have been writing about pain or darkness. Call it synchronicity, perhaps. Call it the Universe or God connecting with me. It matters not to me what your take is on that. All I ask is that you remain open.

As for myself, I feel no need to question. For it is as it is, and things are as they are. I openly choose to share with you what is happening for me right here, right now: The wind is still gently blowing the leaves in the trees around me. It feels as if the wind and trees are speaking directly to me. I hear those same words again, but now even louder: 'Grow, Maureen, grow.' I am going to stop writing for a bit—I have goosebumps. I will sit quietly and enjoy the warmth of the summer sun for a sacred space as stillness is growing and emerging within me.

LIFE IS FOR CERTAIN AN EDUCATIONAL, MAGICAL, MYSTERIOUS PROCESS—A PRIVILEGE OF OUR BIRTHRIGHT AND A GIFT.

Life is for certain an educational, magical, mysterious process—a privilege of our birthright and a gift.

Keeping Things Simple: We do not always need to understand everything in life. There are times it is best to accept. It just is.

RISE: VALUE YOUR BIRTHRIGHT

You change the world by being yourself.

—Yoko Ono

Today's assignment is to read the following commitment aloud. If it resonates with you and you are ready, add your signature and date in the space below.

> Today, I choose to embrace the magic and mystery of life as it unfolds for me. I commit to living my life more fully, doing and being more, and doing all I can to honour the privilege of my birthright. I am of value to this world. I am enough. I am worthy and deserving. When I cannot change my circumstances, I can grow and evolve within them. From this day forwards, I choose to rise and embrace and serve the truth of me.

Signed . . . .

Today's Date . . . .

DAY 14
INVITE POSSIBILITY AND PURPOSE

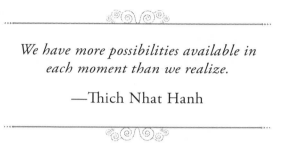

*We have more possibilities available in
each moment than we realize.*

—Thich Nhat Hanh

Possibilities

1. different things that you can do in a particular
   situation

2. opportunities to develop in a successful, interesting,
   or exciting way

3. capability of existing, happening or being true

—Definitions sourced from 1) Oxford Learner's Dictionaries,
2) Macmillan Dictionary, and
3) WordWeb Online Dictionary and Thesaurus.

***In a Nutshell: Possibilities present various opportunities
for you to make happen or achieve.***

If you were to meet me in person, it might appear to you that I am a wounded warrior. At a superficial level, my physical body or life may not seem rewarding or good. I use a wheelchair outdoors and need help at home. I live on a liquid diet. My muscles are atrophied, and my body looks frail and weak.

But do not let that fool you—I am emotionally and spiritually stronger than I have ever been.

Through my own experiences and pain, life has given me the golden key to access something deeply special that others may never get the opportunity to know or discover. You too have that opportunity. At the core of your current pain and challenges, you have a wealth of opportunities for personal growth.

Yes—your situation may seem bleak to you. Your pain and illness may be challenging and ever-present. The meaning of life, however, is the personal meaning you put to it. What matters most is what you think now, what you see in your mind now, what direction you choose to steer those pictures you are making, and how you shape your thoughts.

> WHAT MATTERS MOST IS WHAT YOU THINK NOW, WHAT YOU SEE IN YOUR MIND NOW, WHAT DIRECTION YOU CHOOSE TO STEER THOSE PICTURES YOU ARE MAKING, AND HOW YOU SHAPE YOUR THOUGHTS.

Let nothing dim the light that shines from within.

—Maya Angelou

INVITE POSSIBILITY AND PURPOSE

The Problem

The problem is that we quickly get used to new ways of living. We adapt to our circumstances and settle into them, even when those circumstances are not our choice and feel uncomfortable. As a result, we become increasingly complacent with our discomfort. We make excuses to ourselves for not trying to improve our lives (often convincing ourselves that our excuses are genuine reasons): things are out of our control, and there is nothing that we can do. We can stop ourselves from seeing the different possibilities available to us. Like a horse with blinders on, we have a limited awareness of what is all around us and develop tunnel vision.

Sadly, this can leave us feeling stuck in a rut; we become used to living each day encased in our discomfort. We neglect daily nourishing practices and our self-care. As a result, our emotional well-being and zest for living can start to spiral down a drab and dreary path.

It is a hard truth, but living in a world of what we feel we have lost or that illness has taken from us will never improve things. On the contrary, it will only prevent us from making the most of the life that is available to us.

Only when we accept our situation as it is and determine to make the most of it do we find the light in the darkness and unwrap the gifts and rewards available to us. Only then do we develop an inner sense of purpose and a growing awareness of the rewarding possibilities our situation brings.

THERE IS NO PURPOSE TOO BIG

If the word *purpose* scares you, or you think that purpose is only for those who are fit and healthy, know that no purpose in life is too big for you. Possibilities abound if you are willing to seek and see them. We may not be able to heal the world, but each of us can play a part. Making a difference does not require you to be fully physically fit and well.

Through your pain and discomfort, you can learn the power of self-love and kindness and the importance of self-care. You can live life with greater purpose and develop more compassion, understanding, patience, and tolerance. You can give and share more love. None of these things would be made so richly available to you in a life free of challenges or a state of constant bliss.

Your pain and wounds have the power to manifest much wisdom—through your personal experiences, you can help others by sharing what you have come to learn and know. In life, you must experience the things you are here to inspire or help others with as you guide, support, or teach.

Keeping Things Simple: Moving through your pain to meaning and purpose is a possibility available to all.

RISE: INVITE POSSIBILITY AND PURPOSE

When you hand good people possibility, they do great things.

—Biz Stone

It is Day 14, and your *Rise* assignment today is to answer the following questions. Take time to explore the possibilities that can help you both live with your pain and positively move through your pain to purpose, greater fulfilment, and a more rewarding life.

Questions to Ask Yourself

In what way might I still be attached to what has happened to me or the conditioned thoughts of who I am?

. . . .
. . . .
. . . .
. . . .

To what extent am I embracing new possibilities as they arise for me in each moment?

. . . .
. . . .
. . . .
. . . .

How can I redirect my thoughts away from the darkness of pain and illness and towards enthusiastically embracing the possibilities available to me?

. . . .
. . . .
. . . .
. . . .

What could I do differently?

. . . .
. . . .
. . . .
. . . .

What do I need to think about anew?

. . . .
. . . .
. . . .
. . . .

How can I move forwards now? What is my next best step?

. . . .
. . . .
. . . .

DAY 15
WELCOME MAGIC AND WONDER

This is a wonderful day. I have never seen this one before.

—Maya Angelou

Day

1. one of the numbered 24-hour periods into which a week, month, or year is divided

2. the period of time, the solar day, during which the earth makes one complete revolution on its axis relative to the sun

3. the time of light between one night and the next

—Definitions sourced from 1) YourDictionary,
2) Dictionary.com, and
3) Merriam-Webster.

In a Nutshell: Day is the time of light between one night and the next which elicits a feeling of wonder.

Today is a new day, and for that, I am so grateful. Yesterday was hard; I spent most of the day curled up under a warmed fleecy blanket on the lounge sofa in a darkened room. My dogs curled up right beside me, doing all they could to hold the calm and space for me and provide compassion in my time of need.

Functioning at a physical level yesterday felt near impossible. It is safe to say that soul-eroding pain did all it could to consume me. The great thing, however, is that it was yesterday. The day that is here right now is a new day and a chance to let yesterday go and start again.

That knowledge brings much comfort. To awaken to a new day, with unique moments unfolding, and to be able to let go of the darkness of yesterday brings fresh, energising freedom. Staying connected to the preciousness of each day is what helps keep me moving positively forwards and fully living life despite having relentless pain and ever-present fatigue as companions.

What is the gift of a new day? And what can it mean to you?

In truth, today is the only day you will ever have that has the power to create a good yesterday for tomorrow. Unfortunately, this day is not available for rerun—it can never return to you for readjustment or replay.

By tomorrow, today will be but a memory, and the stark reality is that you and I are both exchanging a day of our lives for today; as the sun goes down each night and the day comes to an end, we have one day less to live on this earth.

As each new morning comes, however, we are presented with a blank page, a page on which we can craft, create, shape, steer, and direct our story. We can let today slip into the mundane and go by in a blur, or we can do as much as we can to live, love, and laugh more. As each day awakens, our souls and spirits are presented with the invitation to rise from slumber and awaken too.

> AS EACH DAY AWAKENS, OUR SOULS AND SPIRITS ARE PRESENTED WITH THE INVITATION TO RISE FROM SLUMBER AND AWAKEN TOO.

And that is somewhat magical, awesome, forgiving, and freeing.

I do not wish the blessings of this day to be stolen by the memories of the overly challenging day I had yesterday. Nor do I want it to be darkened by worrying or stressing needlessly about what the rest of my week will bring. I will take one day at a time, and as each new dawn breaks, I will do all I can to breathe in fresh courage, renewed mental resilience, a strengthened spirit, deeper inner peace, more steadfast hope, and greater calm and comfort.

As the saying goes, if you smile at life, it is more likely to smile at you.

When you awaken to the preciousness of each day and fully take it on board, you start to feel so much more inspired to make each day a little less ordinary—you find yourself fuelled by gratitude and appreciation of your Creator's gift.

Let us get real. This does not mean that you will not have days when you feel physically rough, and things may get on top of you. It does not mean that you will not feel mentally low at times, emotionally challenged, or exhausted by your plight.

Every morning, however, stands for hope. It gives you another chance at life and presents an opportunity to embrace the new day more fully.

Yesterday is history. Tomorrow is a mystery. Today is a gift.

—Eleanor Roosevelt

Keeping Things Simple: Echoing the words of Marty Robbins, 'Every day is a good day to be alive whether the sun's shining or not.'[8]

RISE: WELCOME MAGIC AND WONDER

*Thank you, dear God, for this good life and
forgive us if we do not love it enough.*

—Garrison Keillor

The day that is your *today* is precious. It is up to you how fully you live it, whether you choose to live it half-heartedly or live it well. We are now on Day 15 and halfway through your elixir, and your *Rise* assignment today is to ask yourself the following questions:

Did I give myself fully to today? (Circle your answer.)

Yes   No

Did I embrace all the opportunities this day offered?

Yes   No

What achievements or actions today am I most proud of myself for?

. . . .

. . . .

. . . .

. . . .

. . . .

. . . .

What might I do differently tomorrow?

. . . .
. . . .
. . . .
. . . .
. . . .
. . . .

What action(s) could I commit to take when I wake up tomorrow to welcome in the new day?

. . . .
. . . .
. . . .
. . . .
. . . .
. . . .

As you move forward, I encourage you to commit to asking yourself these same questions every evening and jotting down your answers in your diary, journal, or notebook so you may reflect on them at a future date.

DAY 16
REST IN GOD

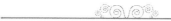

Rest is not some holy feeling that comes upon us in church. It is a state of calm rising from a heart deeply and firmly established in God.

—Henry Drummond

God

1. the Being perfect in power, wisdom, and goodness who is worshipped as creator and ruler of the universe

2. a spirit or being believed to control some part of the universe or life and often worshiped for doing so, or something that represents this spirit or being

3. source of all moral authority; the supreme being

—Definitions sourced from 1) Merriam-Webster, 2) Cambridge Dictionary, and 3) Lexico Dictionaries.

In a Nutshell: God is an image, person, or entity that you believe to be the Creator of the Universe and world in which you live.

As I opened the book *Streams in the Desert* this morning to read the entry for today's date, the words from Psalm 23 stood out for me. As J. Hudson Taylor highlights in the February 8 entry, Psalm 23 does not say the Lord *was* my shepherd or that he *will be* my shepherd. It does not say he *may be* my shepherd or that he *can be*. It simply states that he *is* my shepherd, and that means he is always here with me right here, right now.

I am a firm believer that each of us, as we go through life, develops an individual and deeply personal relationship with a Higher Power and that it matters not what you choose to call that presence. Therefore, whether you choose to name that presence God, Supreme Creator, or some other name you are comfortable with, is not what is important. In truth, I do not think God would mind or be upset if you referred to him by a different term or name. What *is* important is that you openly welcome his presence in your life.

Despite the tidal wave of exhaustion which is doing its best to consume me this morning and the fiery dragon of pain raising its ugly head, challenging my every movement, I take rest in knowing that my God is here.

And that brings me much comfort—for it means I am not alone on life's journey.

HE IS ALWAYS HERE WITH ME RIGHT HERE, RIGHT NOW.

I am supported.

I am guided.

The Lord is my shepherd.

—Psalm 23:1

A Relationship Is a Two-Way Thing

Spiritual people are not those who engage in certain spiritual practices; they are those who draw their life from a conversational relationship with God.

—Dallas Willard

I openly speak, and I ask. I create and hold the space to listen and hear—and he answers. I invite his words to enter, and I reflect on them. And then, with soul stripped and open, I respond.

That is the thing about communication—communication is always a two-way thing. Having a relationship with God is no different from any other relationship—whether that be a relationship between a husband and wife, a parent and child, one colleague or friend and another, a teacher with a pupil, a doctor or nurse with a patient, and so forth. Relationships, to be real relationships, require communication and interaction with all participants playing their equal parts.

There Is Little to Be Gained

There is no point in asking for God's support or help if you are not prepared to create the time and space within your day's bustle and busyness to open your heart, mind, and ears to hear his answer.

There is no point in praying to the Universe to help make something happen for you if you are not willing to open your awareness to all that is happening around you and recognise the opportunities when they are present.

Living a spiritual life is never all about receiving and taking. Living as a soul alive on earth is not about sitting back as the silent partner expecting magic or miracles to happen.

In life, we must be willing to be raw and vulnerable. No matter our circumstances, we must be prepared to step up to life, interact with it, develop a working relationship with the Supreme Creator, and be wholly committed to living well and taking responsibility for our unique role in the Universe.

Keeping Things Simple: Finding rest in God, and developing a relationship with God, is there for all and a choice you can make.

RISE: REST IN GOD

The truth is—you are as close to God as you choose to be.

—Rick Warren

For your assignment today, I encourage you to think about God and the quality of how you interact together.

Do you speak?

Do you create quiet and space for your voice to be heard? And to listen to his answer?

What action(s) do you think you could take now to further your spiritual growth and enrich your place of rest within?

. . . .

. . . .

. . . .

. . . .

. . . .

. . . .

. . . .

. . . .

. . . .

. . . .

. . . .

. . . .

. . . .

DAY 17
HOLD ON TO FAITH

*Faith is the bird that feels the light
when the dawn is still dark.*

—Rabindranath Tagore

Faith

1. great trust or confidence in something or someone

2. firm belief in something for which there is no proof

3. the substance of things hoped for, the evidence of things not seen

> —Definitions sourced from 1) Cambridge Dictionary,
> 2) Merriam-Webster, and
> 3) Hebrews 11:1.

In a Nutshell: Faith is complete confidence and trust in a person, concept, or thing.

I never cease to be amazed by all the different colours and shades of green visible in the trees, shrubs, and flowers in my garden. There are so many varying depths and hues—from light to dark, soft to bold, gracefully feminine and gentle to vivid, masculine, and strong.

Life is the same. It is a mixed bag of events, situations, and circumstances presenting us with various depths and shades of emotions. Being fully alive to life means being alive to all it offers us—whether our life is coloured with black or white, different shades of grey, or peppered with a rainbow of experiences or events.

When pain does its best to consume me, I take great strength from spending time in nature and looking at the trees. In the challenges of winter and barren of leaves, they appear vulnerable—raw, real, and naked. And yet they do not appear defeated; they still stand strong. They are courageous. They remain trusting and faithful. Grounded in their strong roots and foundations and connected to their very core being, the trees seem to know that the harshness of the winter months will pass and new growth will come when spring and summer emerge, as Mother Nature intended. As they stand bare and unprotected from the harsh elements, the trees redirect their focus and energy inwards to do all they can to restore their strength so that when the brighter days and nights come, they can burst forth renewed and awakened. The winters of their life are natural components necessary for their well-being and growth.

As spirits and souls on earth, having a human experience, our life events and circumstances present us with that same opportunity for growth. It is only through letting our Creator work through us in our times of darkness and difficulties that our faith can be fully birthed, exercised, developed, and increased.

Real faith is trusting, not only when things are going well but even when you are feeling troubled, uncomfortable, overwhelmed, rejected, or discouraged. Real faith means having faith even when you are living in the dark and do not understand your God's plan.

> REAL FAITH MEANS HAVING FAITH EVEN WHEN YOU ARE LIVING IN THE DARK AND DO NOT UNDERSTAND YOUR GOD'S PLAN.

Faith is the strength by which a shattered world shall emerge into the light.

—Helen Keller

PRAYER IS NOT ENOUGH ON ITS OWN

The universe does not hear what you are saying. It feels the vibration you are offering.

—Abraham Hicks

With a growing faith often comes a natural increase in chatting with God and praying. Prayers need not be overcomplicated, clever, or long. All that is important is that they come from a heartfelt place.

You must *feel the words* you are saying, singing, or writing and offer them with belief, trust, and knowing that your prayers will be answered in the Universe's perfect timing and in God's perfect way. Without feeling the vibration of belief and faith underlying your words, they will remain nothing more than words. For the power of prayer to be released, you must fully connect with your words—you must offer them freely, wholly, and unconditionally.

Be patient. Believe and know that with increasing faith and trust, God will not only *hear* your prayer but in divine timing he will *answer*.

Keeping Things Simple: The power of prayer can only be released when rising faith is behind it. It is up to you to seed your faith firmly so that it can develop strong roots and grow.

RISE: HOLD ON TO FAITH

*Accept what is, let go of what was, and
have faith in what will be.*

—Sonia Ricotti

Asking for help does not always come easy. We can put up protective barriers around ourselves and perceive asking for help from others as a sign of shortcomings and weakness. Whatever your religious or spiritual beliefs may have been until now, all I ask is that you remain open and curious. Awakening the power of faith and prayer is simple. Today's assignment is to insert the words of your choosing below:

God, I ask:

. . . .

. . . .

. . . .

. . . .

. . . .

. . . .

. . . .

. . . .

. . . .

. . . .

. . . .

. . . .

PART FOUR

ENLIVEN

Life's experiences will just keep repeating themselves unless you continually add some new experiences to enliven your days.

—Steven Redhead

DAY 18
OWN YOUR SPACE

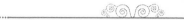

Everyone needs to be able to have their own space in which to be themselves.

—Emily Osment

Space

1. the freedom to live, think, and develop in a way that suits one

2. the opportunity to assert or experience one's identity or needs freely

3. an area of business in which a person or an organization operates

> —Definitions sourced from 1) Lexico Dictionaries,
> 2) Merriam-Webster, and
> 3) Oxford Learner's Dictionaries.

In a Nutshell: Space is the three-dimensional area around you in which you operate and live.

On Day 17, we talked about the benefits of living with faith. It would be best if you took on board, however, the fact that faith does not work on its own. You cannot sit back and expect the Universe or God to deliver all the answers to your problems without you playing your part. You must be prepared to take responsibility for your place and space in the world. You must take ownership of your decisions, choices, and actions. It is up to you to find the calm in your chaos, quieten your storms, and know how to access the safe place inside of you when at a superficial or physical level things may feel soul or spirit dampening, downright difficult, or turbulent. What you let into your world will impact who you are. The space you create around you and what you allow to feed your soul, spirit, and mind shapes the world you live in and shapes and creates *you*.

I was still water, held by my surroundings. I
am now a river carving my own path.

—Scott Stabile

SOUL ~~SURVIVAL~~ THRIVAL

As with all things in life, you have a choice. You can surround yourself with a space that erodes your soul and enthusiasm for life, or you can consciously choose your inputs to uplift and nourish you and positively benefit you in some way.

Put simply, what you take in shapes what you put out; your inputs will impact your outputs. The space you create around you will subconsciously make and influence you and how you show up in your world.

For your soul to become Unhackable and thrive, no matter your health challenges or circumstances, you must be responsible for who or what you let take your soul's attention and what messages you permit to feed you. You can settle for a day-to-day hamster wheel existence in a world that maintains your space of pain and illness—or you can consciously let enter what empowers and enlivens your soul, maintains its wellness, and vitalizes your spirit to rise and soar.

CHOOSE YOUR INPUTS

Motivational quotes that nourish and uplift me surround me in my office. Bright, inspiring prints and pictures cover the wall. A painting of a soaring bird reminds me about freedom of spirit and an image of a goldfish jumping out of a glass bowl reminds me that we have no limitations to what we think we can achieve.

A small silver ornament on my desk reminds me that peace and contentment are found within me. There is also an ornament of a singing bird to remind me that no matter how dark the night, the birds always sing in the morning. A vase of fresh flowers serves to remind me of the impermanence of life and the joy to be found in the beauty of nature. A tube of hand cream prompts me to be intentional about self-care. Bright, colourful stationery and pens, several beautifully scented candles, and many personal development books and journals line the shelves simply because I like them.

In my office, you will find nothing relating to my pain and illness—nothing would take away, detract, infiltrate, or disturb my positive enthusiasm for life or risk depleting my soul. Even the coaster that my coffee cup is sitting on states the words *Be Happy*. I wear a ring on my finger that the designer named 'Wings of Freedom'.

There is also a small gift bag sitting within sight of my desk on top of my filing cabinet with a beautifully wrapped present for myself for when I complete the draft manuscript of this book. The present to me has a gift label with the handwritten words, 'Well done! You did it! With much love from me to you.' The present itself, my reward to me, is a silver necklace engraved with the words 'she believed she could, and so she did'. That necklace is my motivation and reward to unwrap when I finally get all the words that want to be written through me onto the page.

Create Touchstones

Touchstones, like the items in my office, are one way to choose what you allow into your mind. Take ownership of what you feed your subconscious. Surround yourself with things that light you up or uplift you in some way. Likewise, be intentional about mixing with people who feel like sunshine.

Own your space and who and what you allow in it. Every day, aim to touch base with some of those soul-nourishing people, events, or things. Whether it is picking some fresh flowers from your garden or having them delivered with your supermarket shopping, buying a new uplifting book or magazine, lighting a scented candle, enjoying the smell of fresh bread from your kitchen, or uploading an inspiring image or quote as the background on your phone or computer, send positive messages to your brain. Do not let the unwanted or unnecessary hack the quality of your thoughts or soul. Make a conscious decision each day to feed your soul what it needs and be willing to go where it needs and wants to go.

> MAKE A CONSCIOUS DECISION EACH DAY TO FEED YOUR SOUL WHAT IT NEEDS AND BE WILLING TO GO WHERE IT NEEDS AND WANTS TO GO.

CHOOSE POSITIVE INPUTS

To create change in your world, you must learn to protect the space you live in and appreciate it. I encourage you to get to know yourself better and do whatever it is that enlivens your mood and empowers your soul and spirit. Walk confidently inside your story and own it. Understand your needs so you can enthusiastically show up to your world wholly and completely. Choose your inputs wisely; create a space that rejuvenates your passion, drive, and energy.

Keeping Things Simple: You become what you surround yourself with. The energies around you are contagious. Choose carefully. Choose wisely. The environment and space you inhabit have the power to craft and shape you.

RISE: OWN YOUR SPACE

*Your environment and the associations you keep will affect how
you think, feel, and act, and ultimately the results you get.*

—Mensah Oteh

Your Day 18 assignment is to take a few moments to look
around you and think about the environment you spend most
of your time in. Jot down which elements of that space provide
nourishing, positive messages. Also note the elements around
you which drain your energy.

Positive Nourishing Inputs

. . . .

. . . .

. . . .

. . . .

. . . .

. . . .

. . . .

. . . .

. . . .

. . . .

Unhelpful or Depleting Inputs

. . . .

. . . .

. . . .

. . . .

. . . .

. . . .

. . . .

. . . .

. . . .

. . . .

Over the next few days and weeks, commit to making small but significant changes to diminish the negative inputs in your life and increase the inputs that motivate, inspire, or uplift you. In addition, commit to taking at least one action to instigate positive change in your personal space within the next twenty-four hours.

DAY 19
CRAFT YOUR CALM

Don't try to calm the storm. Calm yourself. The storm will pass.

—Timber Hawkeye

Calm

1. not affected by strong emotions such as excitement, anger, shock, or fear

2. without drama . . . a state of peace or stillness

3. to soothe and pacify; not excited or agitated; composed

—Definitions sourced from 1) Macmillan Dictionary,
2) Vocabulary.com, and
3) YourDictionary.

In a Nutshell: Calm is peace and steadiness of mind under stress.

No matter how much you take ownership of your own space, there will be times when the pain tsunamis hit. The seas will roil no matter how uplifting and inspiring the environment you have created. In truth, all the personal touchstones you have now placed around your home to enhance your self-esteem and positive feelings will need some help if you have any chance of keeping afloat when powerful drama, pain flares, and crises hit. You risk drowning in your chaos unless you learn to find calm in your storms. When you feel you have no energy or power to calm the storm, you must craft calm in *you* until the storm's ferocity passes.

I experienced this for myself when I was out in Los Angeles in 2017 for specialist medical treatment. I had travelled from Scotland to undergo two complex surgeries scheduled only two weeks apart. The first surgery went well, and for the most part, I felt on top of things. Dr Gelabert was highly skilled and wonderfully supportive and helped make sure I was as comfortable as could be expected with the invasive procedures my body was going through.

The second surgery, however, took its toll. Two weeks to the day after having my first rib removed and pectoral and scalene muscles stripped back on the right side of my chest, I was in the operating theatre for the same procedures to be carried out on my left side. I awoke several hours later in the recovery room engulfed in a fierce fire of pain that would not subside despite the pain consultants' best efforts. I was caught in the eye of the storm, and the barrage was relentless. A sense of overwhelm gripped my mind and body. I felt physically and mentally sabotaged, consumed in a storm I could not escape.

After I was discharged from the hospital and back in our rented apartment several days later, the fiery storm showed no signs of abating. Pain and total exhaustion engulfed me. The storm's turbulence proved near impossible to calm, so I had no option but to find calm *within* the storm, redirect my focus to the safe place within me, and take steps to calm myself.

You must learn to do the same if you do not want to be engulfed by your pain flares and crises. When pain overtakes you and fiercely raises its intensity, you must learn to let go of your attention to it, reach inside, gather all the broken pieces of trauma, pull them into your heart and soul, and infuse them with your love, compassion, and kindness. You must listen and let go of what no longer serves you well, slow down and breathe, and drop into the stillness within you and into your safe place. You must learn techniques to tame your pain and change the way your brain sees your pain. You must get to know yourself better, understand your needs at a deeper level, and be willing and prepared to figure out how to best support yourself.

You fortify what you focus on—so you must learn to take your attention away from the assault on your physical body and redirect your attention. When you consciously and consistently drop down to the still and calm of your soul and spirit, you will find a safe place to find rest and shelter until the height of the storm passes.

Life is like a river. Sometimes it sweeps you gently along and sometimes the rapids come out of nowhere.

—Emma Smith

Smooth Seas Never Make Skilled Sailors

Storms often draw something out of us that calm seas don't.

—Bill Hybels

When you feel caught up in the storm and think life is unfair, know that without experiencing the highest of highs in life and the lowest of lows, the depth of emotions you feel would likely remain unchanged. It would be difficult for you to differentiate between joy and boredom, between pain and comfort, between anxiety and calm, between dark and light, and between love and hate. Everything would bring you the same depth of feelings. Good, bad, or indifferent; black, grey, or white would appear and feel the same.

The most meaningful things in life are often brought to your attention through challenging times as well as good times. Both ends of the spectrum can offer significant learning opportunities if you open your eyes, mind, and heart to their gifts. There is truth in the saying 'A calm sea has never made a skilled sailor'. When you cannot calm the storm, remember to access the safe and calm within you. Learn all you can from the storm and let it teach you how to be a stronger person.

WHEN YOU CANNOT CALM THE STORM, REMEMBER TO ACCESS THE SAFE AND CALM WITHIN YOU.

127

Echoing the wisdom of Ben Greenhalgh, 'No matter how strong the storm, how hard the rain and how vicious the wind there is always a gap in the clouds for the light to shine through.'[9]

VISUALISATION TECHNIQUES TO HELP CALM YOURSELF IN THE STORM

We can weather anything if we stay calm in the eye of the storm.

—Lolly Daskal

I shared a relaxing and calming breathing exercise with you on Day 9 and touched on the power of meditation. Sometimes, however, the intensity of your pain can hack your ability to take ownership of your breathing pattern and drop down into the safe place within your body to create some solitude and space.

The following visualisation and self-hypnosis techniques may be something new to you, and you may even think that they are a bit 'woo-woo' or that I am belittling the severity of your pain. I urge you not to discount these practices without trying them. They can be an empowering addition to the pain management techniques you may already use. Furthermore, at a personal level, I find them a godsend when my body is experiencing severe pain flares.

Start by directing your focus to where the pain is at its worst intensity in your body and envisage that pain as being a specific shape and colour. It may be that you see it as a fiery red star, jagged black square or triangle, pulsating orange ball, green oval, purple-spotted rectangle, or something else. (Take ownership of this visualisation; there is no right or wrong. Your pain is your personal experience. Do not overthink this one—picture a shape and colour that comes to mind and seems to best connect with your pain and go with that.)

VISUALISATION OPTION #1

Consciously change the shape and colour of the pain you have seen in your mind into something completely different, e.g., change the image of your jagged red star to a pale pink circle or your sharp black triangle to a soft green square. You will alter how your brain perceives your pain by adjusting the way your brain sees and relays the physical sensations your body is going through.

VISUALISATION OPTION #2

After envisioning your pain as something with a specific shape and colour, imagine taking that coloured shape in its totality from your body into your hand. Direct your full focus and attention onto it, clench your fist around it—and then in your mind proceed to throw it (physically making the movement of throwing a ball) far off into the distance or to smack against a faraway wall. The farther you distance and separate yourself in your mind from your pain, the less discomfort you will feel.

If you have a supportive family member or friend who is willing to help, you can take this technique a step further.

I demonstrated the following steps in a pain management workshop with a lady named Ella whose knee pain was so intense it was proving near impossible for her to concentrate or join in. Noticing Ella's severe discomfort, I asked her to focus on seeing and naming her pain as a shape and a colour, then to visualise taking that pain out of her knee and carefully placing it into the palm of my open hand.

And that was when the magic happened: with her pain now in my possession, Ella watched as I started to walk away from her, and the farther I walked, the less discomfort she told me she was feeling. When I took a couple of steps closer towards her again (still with her pain in my hand and offering to give it back to her), she said, 'I cannot believe what you are doing to me. My pain is coming back! This is unbelievable. This is so weird!'

As I started to distance myself from her again, Ella confirmed her pain levels were once more diminishing. Seeing an opportunity to give Ella even greater relief, I proceeded to 'throw her pain' out of an open window and told her to relax and enjoy the rest of the workshop as her pain was now outside amid some dense bushes some six or eight feet below. As if a magician had popped up and announced *abracadabra*, Ella told me the severe pain in her knee had now greatly subsided, and was, for the most part, gone.

What I did that day was not to magically heal and free Ella of her ongoing health condition and discomfort. Much as I would have loved to give her permanent relief from her severe arthritis, I had not demonstrated or manifested a miracle healing cure. I had helped Ella provide the message to her brain that the pain was outside of her, now over there, and out the window. I provided the opportunity for her to refocus her attention elsewhere, breathe in fresh energy, recuperate, and rest.

Call it 'hocus pocus' if you like; I can understand that. When I was first introduced to this technique, I was highly sceptical and blocked myself from trying it for quite some time.

VISUALISATION OPTION #3

If you have trouble sleeping or resting because of your pain, a softer and more gradual way of adjusting your brain's perception of your discomfort can often help gently guide you into a more deeply relaxed state.

As before, envisage the area of your most severe pain as being of a specific shape and colour (and hold an image of that in your mind). Once you have that, redirect your focus and attention to a part of your body that feels more comfortable and see it as having its own appropriate softer or brighter colour.

Now, imagine a paintbrush in your hand, dip the paintbrush into that more comfortable colour, see the brush fully loaded with that specific colour, and visualise painting over the previously envisioned colour and shape of your worst pain. Start by softening any hard or jagged edges. Then keep going back and forth (dipping your paintbrush back into the colour of your more comfortable body area as often as you need) until you have completely shaded over your focused image of pain. You will find you have successfully lessened your discomfort by painting it the same colour as the area of your body which your brain perceives to be much more comfortable or pain-free.

Keeping Things Simple: Taking steps to alter how your brain sees and perceives pain can change the experience of how you feel the pain. Visualisation is a powerful technique to have in your pain management toolkit, and like anything, it takes practice. However, the more you practise, the easier it will become for you, and the more effective and beneficial it will prove to be.

RISE: CRAFT YOUR CALM

*The closer a man comes to a calm mind
the closer he is to strength.*

—Marcus Aurelius

Your Day 19 *Rise* assignment is to pull up a picture in your mind of an occasion, time, or place when you have felt deeply at peace with the world, content, calm, or relaxed. If pain has consumed you as of late and you struggle to think of a specific time, imagine yourself in a situation as relaxed and comfortable as you would ideally like to be.

Visualise yourself experiencing the same relaxed emotions and feelings as if you were in that same place now.

Allow yourself to soak up and enjoy those feelings, shut your eyes—and imagine holding them deep within you.

When you open your eyes, bring those same feelings with you as you gently ease into your present moment and move forwards with your day.

Day 20
PRACTISE SELF-CARE

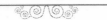

An empty lantern provides no light. Self-care is the fuel that allows your light to shine brightly.

—Author Unknown

Self-Care

1. the practice of taking action to preserve or improve one's own health

2. doing activities to take care of your mental, emotional, and physical health

3. the practice of activities that are necessary to sustain life and health, normally initiated and carried out by the individual for him- or herself

—Definitions sourced from 1) Lexico Dictionaries,
2) The Summit Counseling Center[10], and
3) Oxford Reference.

In a Nutshell: Self-care is engaging in activities and practices to nurture and maintain the health and well-being of your mind, body, spirit, and soul.

Caring well for yourself is your responsibility in life. It relies on you being aware and attentive to your own emotional, physical, and spiritual needs and consciously answering those needs as best as you can.

There are no set rules when it comes to self-care. You do not have to follow a particular diet, be a vegan, practise yoga, go to church, or spend hours staring at the stars and moon, exercising, meditating, or polishing your physical body. What self-care does mean, however, is taking care of your mind and thoughts; your physical, emotional, and spiritual health; your moods, energy, and emotions; and listening to and honouring the deepest needs of what lies within your core and soul.

You are your own healer. You have the power to influence what will happen for you. It's work that you need to do.

—Michael Finkelstein, MD

Be Clear

Self-care is not about being self-indulgent, nor is it selfish. It is something that feeds, nourishes, and fuels you. It should never deplete you. It is about respecting yourself and doing all you can to enhance and maintain your holistic well-being and minimising your feelings of discomfort, emotional or physical turmoil, anxiety, or stress. Neither should self-care ever be an emergency response action only practised in times of crisis. Self-care is an ongoing personal journey and relies on developing and honouring a growing awareness of your own ever-evolving mind/body/spirit/soul needs.

Although a simple concept, *you* taking care of *you* is often not prioritised. It is all too easy to concentrate on looking after everyone else in your family first or to be so consumed by your discomfort that you overlook nurturing your health and well-being.

DON'T KNOW WHERE TO START?

There is no need to feel overwhelmed at the prospect of looking after yourself better. It is best to simply start where you are and commit to making small nourishing changes to your ways of caring for yourself, thinking, acting, being, and doing. Paying attention to your nutrition and quality of sleep, maintaining regular, gentle exercise (as you are physically able to do so), and ensuring adequate periods of relaxation are all intrinsic elements contributing to your overall feelings of well-being. It is equally important not to neglect the continuous enrichment of your mind, spirit, and soul—where your true power lies. Looking after your soul and mind and breathing the fire of passion into all you do is what will free your healing medicine to do its best job.

For me, there is no doubt that writing releases my soul-healing medicine. There is a *me* that arises within it and emerges—and I do not always need to write much or write well. It never fails to be my food and fuel, enabling me to gently coax my emotions and thoughts away from my pain and guide them in a more beneficial direction. Writing is my caring, compassionate companion that takes my hand

and comforts me, even in my most difficult challenges, pain flares, and change.

We are all born creative beings. We are not inanimate objects meant to stay static, waiting for life to happen. Our souls need a creative outlet to release the comforting presence of the vitalizing power of life that lies within.

As I let myself write now, my pain no longer demands my attention in the same way. The full force of the raging fire in my nerves and bones is starting to soften ever so subtly. I am not naïve—the war is not over. My pain continues—but I have consciously and positively guided and steered my attention away from it. I am in the throes of successfully metabolizing my pain as positive, creative energy and purpose.

I find myself smiling on the inside.

My healing medicine is doing its job.

You Must Discover Your Healing Medicine

We *all* need to discover our own healing medicine—no matter what illness or disability we have, the source of our pain, or how our personal experience of pain affects us. We all deserve to discover that powerful potion that makes a meaningful difference to us, touches us, frees us, enables us to soften our discomfort with life, and transforms us at our core.

It is not simply about having something that distracts you for a while. Having something you can commit yourself to will lift and nourish you at a fulfilling and rewarding deep soul level. When your pain risks closing in on you, you must take responsibility and ownership to shift your mind, body, spirit, and soul to a different place.

It does not mean that your pain will not exist anymore. What it will mean is that you are choosing to lead your attention elsewhere to something that will trigger and ignite better emotions and feelings for you instead.

Unlike traditional medication issued to you on prescription by your doctor, the brilliant thing is that this form of healing medicine comes with no risk of adverse side effects. On the contrary, *feel excited.* The benefits of practising soul-care are spirit-lifting and huge.

A Timely Tip

You do not need to feel a bit better or have a better day or a better week before you start putting your soul's self-care higher up your list of priorities. It is not helpful to put your self-care on hold or only half-heartedly participate in it whilst you wait in the hope of your doctor producing a new miracle medication or other medical professionals waving their magic wand. It is important simply to *start where you are* to take better care of yourself and consciously and consistently make small changes from there.

> IT IS IMPORTANT SIMPLY TO START WHERE YOU ARE TO TAKE BETTER CARE OF YOURSELF AND CONSCIOUSLY AND CONSISTENTLY MAKE SMALL CHANGES FROM THERE.

An Unhackable Soul is a soul that is secure and strong.

A soul alive is a soul you have ignited.

A soul on fire is one whose light you keep burning brightly.

They say God best helps those who carry out the work they need to do to best help themselves.

Keeping Things Simple: Practising self-care at a mind/body/spirit/soul holistic level is a form of self-leadership which involves making conscious choices and decisions about how and where you want to show up in life. If you are going to squeeze more comfort and joy from life, it is work you need to do.

RISE: PRACTISE SELF-CARE

*Self care means giving the world the best of
you instead of what is left of you.*

—Katie Reed

Your body, mind, spirit, and soul cannot play their best part
in your life if you do not look after them well and feed and
nourish them regularly. For today's assignment, grab a pen or
pencil, and in the space below, list ten ways you could start
taking better overall care of *you*.

1 . . . .
. . . .

2 . . . .
. . . .

3 . . . .
. . . .

4 . . . .
. . . .

5 . . . .
. . . .

6 . . . .
. . . .

7 . . . .
. . . .

8 . . . .

. . . .

9 . . . .

. . . .

10 . . . .

. . . .

Once you have completed your list, choose one of those things and do it now.

DAY 21
ENLIVEN YOUR SENSES

While you are upon earth, enjoy the good things that are here.

—John Selden

Here

1. in, at, or to this place or position

2. in the present life or state : on earth

3. in the present life or condition

—Definitions sourced from 1) Lexico Dictionaries,
2) Merriam-Webster, and
3) American Heritage Dictionary.

In a Nutshell: Here refers to this time you live now on this earth: in this present time and state.

B e clear: it is not your fault if your soul has felt depleted as of late. Be clear on this also: it is not your fault if you have let your self-care slip for a while or have been feeling somewhat disillusioned with life. The twenty-first-century world can often feel demanding, stressful, or busy. Living in this world is not always easy, and having chronic illness and pain only amplifies that truth. You can become so downtrodden by your pain and discomfort that life can feel downright difficult. Joy can seem like a distant memory. You can start to live in a hazy bubble—or at the other extreme, become so focused on going places and achieving things that you can inadvertently miss out on the richness and beauty that is all around you.

Whilst you are *here* on this earth, you owe it to yourself to be *here* fully.

To richly experience life, you must live it with awakened senses.

Let me share with you a couple of true stories. The first story is about a busker at a Metro station and the second is a personal story of my trip to Bristol. Both stories highlight the importance of living with your senses alive and open.

> WHILST YOU ARE HERE ON THIS EARTH, YOU OWE IT TO YOURSELF TO BE HERE FULLY.

> *Still round the corner there may wait*
> *a new road or a secret gate.*
>
> —J.R.R. Tolkien

The Busker at the Metro: The True Story of Joshua Bell

The earth has music for those who listen.

—Author Unknown

In 2007, as part of an experiment initiated by *Washington Post* columnist Gene Weingarten, premier violinist and Grammy-winning musician Joshua Bell went busking for a full forty-five minutes in a Washington D.C. Metro station. It was at one of their busiest times of day on a cold January morning—commuter rush hour.

Only one person recognised Joshua out of the thousands who passed him that morning, and only seven people stopped to listen to him playing for more than a minute. In total, he earned somewhere in the region of thirty-two dollars.

Joshua is one of the world's greatest musicians and normally preforms on great concert stages. Only two days earlier, he had played the exact same repertoire to a sell-out audience at a theatre in Boston with tickets for his performance costing one hundred dollars each on average.

Interestingly, the person who paid most attention to his performance in the Metro was a three-year-old girl who kept trying to look back to see and hear more. Her mother, focused on her destination, hurried ahead, dragging the little girl along.

The Story of What a Young French Couple Missed

The real voyage of discovery consists not in seeking new landscapes but in having new eyes.

—Marcel Proust

In June 2017, I travelled from Scotland to Bristol for a specialised hospital appointment. I arrived a few hours early and had some time to explore the city, so I took the opportunity to visit Bristol's stunning cathedral. After looking around, I wandered towards the cathedral gardens to enjoy a seat in the summer sun.

The beautiful gardens felt peaceful. I could not help but want to capture the moment and took out a pen and notebook from my handbag. I wrote the following words that morning. When I connect with the feeling these words bring me, I can still imagine I am there now.

> Warmth and light of the golden sun radiating down upon me, pointing straight at me as if it only exists for me—flushing my cheeks, radiating through my chest wall, and warming my soul.

> Traffic noise in the distance, yet not breaking the perfect calm and stillness. Cherry blossom tree standing in all its splendour, protective arms outstretched—a mix of masculine strength and resilience, weaving effortlessly with feminine softness and beauty, bending, flexing, swaying in the gentle breeze with delicate pink fairy-like petals bowing their heads, dancing, and curtsying, with seamless ease and grace.

Vibrant shades of green, a myriad of hues and colours, gently swaying soldier stalks with button moon faces flowing, faces stretched upwards towards the sun.

Peace of tombstones, feeling sacred, savouring an over-whelming sense of deep inner peace.

Birds singing, high-pitched chattering insects hovering and playfully dancing around the verdant bushes.

A weeping willow silhouetted against the clear blue sky, branches bowing as if in prayer, marrying the most beautiful and perfect union of heaven and earth.

About twenty minutes earlier, I had spent a few moments chatting to a young French couple who told me they were on honeymoon and having the trip of a lifetime—a month-long tour of Europe. They told me they were greatly impressed by the cathedral's stunning architecture. When I mentioned I was about to head out to the gardens, however, they told me, 'It's just a graveyard out there. I wouldn't bother. It was quite disappointing. There is nothing much there to see.'

Keeping Things Simple: Your personal experience of each moment is your personal experience. Your world can only ever be as rich and rewarding as you allow it to be.

RISE: ENLIVEN YOUR SENSES

Smell the sea, and feel the sky, let your soul and spirit fly.

—Van Morrison

Today's assignment is to look around you and notice *what you notice*. Then allow your focus and senses complete freedom to go where they naturally want to go. Jot down below what you see, hear, taste, touch, savour, and feel all around:

. . . .

. . . .

. . . .

. . . .

. . . .

. . . .

. . . .

. . . .

. . . .

. . . .

. . . .

. . . .

. . . .

. . . .

. . . .

Now expand your awareness and consciously see, hear, taste, touch, savour, feel, and notice more. Jot down below what you are now aware of that you had not noticed before.

. . . .

. . . .

. . . .

. . . .

. . . .

. . . .

. . . .

. . . .

. . . .

. . . .

. . . .

. . . .

. . . .

. . . .

. . . .

DAY 22
FIND JOY IN THE JOURNEY

The Joy We seek, Can Only Be Created
From The Joy We Have Within.

—Eleesha

Joy

1. a feeling of great happiness

2. the emotion of great delight

3. a settled state of contentment, confidence and hope

   —Definitions sourced from 1) Oxford Learner's Dictionaries,
   2) Dictionary.com, and
   3) Theopedia.

In a Nutshell: Joy is a state of mind and orientation of the heart wrapped in comfort, delight, and peace.

As you start to notice more of the beauty in the world around you, you will find yourself smiling more and, yes, even laughing more. You will discover that you can enjoy life again, both the small and big things—the mundane and, at the other extreme, the wonderful. As you gradually reawaken to life, your more joyous outlook will become evident to those you share your life with. That is okay!

Although it may surprise others to see a smile on your face when they know you are living with ongoing pain and illness, it is okay for you to feel and show happiness, and it is most definitely okay to express your heartfelt joy for life. Experiencing and expressing joy, in fact, will make your happiness deeper. Joy is the fruit that brings meaning and purpose to your life and awakens *you* to life.

> JOY IS THE FRUIT THAT BRINGS MEANING AND PURPOSE TO YOUR LIFE AND AWAKENS YOU TO LIFE.

Joy is what you discover deep within when you strip back all your preconceived ideas of who you are or should be and of what your life could or should look like. Joy is who you are when you let go of all your learned behaviours and mental conditioning and experience the wonder of the world again as if for the first time.

Joy *is* you and an expression of the divine *with* and *within you*. The rich outcome manifests from an ever-growing awareness of the beauty of the world around you, mindful moment-by-moment living, and from you taking personal ownership and responsibility for lighting your darkness. It is the inner delight that evolves from the ever-deepening relationship between you, your world, the Universe, and God.

*Find a place inside where there is joy, and
the joy will burn out the pain.*

—Joseph Campbell

JOY IN THE FACE OF ADVERSITY

It is important to understand that living with joy does not necessarily mean you will not experience adversity. Likewise, living with joy does not mean you will never feel acute sadness, experience grief, or be overwhelmed by loss or pain.

No matter how difficult life may feel, however, each moment holds the possibility to unwrap or discover a joy that rests securely within you. Like happiness, joy does not depend on your circumstances. Joy is the light that you choose to emanate and shine from within you—outwardly to your world—expressing your heartfelt appreciation of life itself and freely embracing your soul and spirit within.

Keeping Things Simple: Living with joy goes much deeper than making the most of things, laughing with friends, or living with a positive outlook. Living with joy means having a deep, meaningful delight in life. It blooms from a secure, sacred place within you.

RISE: FIND JOY IN THE JOURNEY

Joy's soul lies in the doing.

—William Shakespeare

To awaken your joy, you must make supportive and uplifting choices. You must live and act in ways that speak clearly to your heart and soul.

Your Day 22 *Rise* assignment is to ask yourself the following questions and capture your thoughts.

In what ways are my current actions and living patterns separating me from the joy that lies within me?

. . . .
. . . .
. . . .
. . . .
. . . .
. . . .
. . . .
. . . .
. . . .
. . . .
. . . .
. . . .
. . . .

What could I start to do differently from now on to craft more joy in my life?

. . . .
. . . .
. . . .
. . . .
. . . .
. . . .
. . . .
. . . .
. . . .
. . . .
. . . .
. . . .
. . . .
. . . .

DAY 23
CHOOSE TO LOVE

Respect yourself, love yourself because there has never been a person like you and there will never be again.

—Osho

Love

1. an intense feeling of affection

2. to like or desire actively : to hold dear

3. The act of caring and giving to someone. Having someone's best interest and well-being as a priority in your life.

—Definitions sourced from 1) YourDictionary,
2) Merriam-Webster, and
3) Urban Dictionary.

In a Nutshell: Love is a strong attraction and warm emotional attachment to someone or something.

The first definition of love in most dictionaries is 'an intense feeling of deep affection'. Taking that definition at face value implies that love is what one feels. Authentic love, however, is not simply a feeling. Love is a deep personal bond, an unconditional act of caring. When it comes to self-love, it is a bond of acceptance and kindness given to the heart, mind, body, and soul—of you, by you.

Love is reflected in what you do, how you treat yourself and others, how you behave and respond to what is happening in the world you live in, and your environment. When you live in a world shared with pain and illness, however, it is all too easy to see yourself as impaired in some way or broken or physically lacking in some shape or form. Sadly, perceiving yourself as less than perfect in some way or 'needing fixed' only makes it easier to hate yourself for what you are not rather than loving yourself for who and what you already are.

> *One word frees us of all the weight and*
> *pain of life: that word is love.*

—Sophocles

THE PROBLEM IS . . .

The problem is it is easier to love yourself when everything is going well in your life—when things are going as planned and everyone around you accepts and likes you. It is not so easy when your life seems to be falling apart, when you feel rejected, or when you feel your body is letting you down. It is often in your biggest struggles (and when you are most in need of love) that you tend to be least accepting and hardest on yourself.

But here is the good news: you do not have to love everything about your life or everything about yourself to start practising self-love and compassion. What happens on the outside of your world or to your physical body does not need to inhibit your self-respect and compassionate care.

> WHAT HAPPENS ON THE OUTSIDE OF YOUR WORLD OR TO YOUR PHYSICAL BODY DOES NOT NEED TO INHIBIT YOUR SELF-RESPECT AND COMPASSIONATE CARE.

THE SECRET TO SELF-LOVE

Loving yourself comes down to accepting yourself as you already are, including any weaknesses, failures, and mistakes. You must have compassion for yourself as a soul and spirit on earth. Self-love is not simply a state of feeling good. It is a state of appreciation for yourself that evolves from consistently practising loving actions that support the wellness and growth of your physical and psychological self, your soul and spirit.

Loving yourself is one of the most important things you can do, and it takes time and practice to learn. Self-love is about respecting yourself, feeling deserving of taking care of your personal needs, and seeing your happiness as important. Self-love comes down to cultivating a loving and healthy relationship with yourself, being your own champion and unconditionally compassionate best friend.

CHOOSE TO LOVE

SELF-LOVE IS NOT BEING SELF-INDULGENT

Let me be clear: when I talk of self-love, I am not talking about being self-absorbed or narcissistic. Nor do I want you to disregard or be disrespectful of others. Self-love means not settling for less than you deserve because you understand and respect your needs. Loving the truth of you is quite different from self-love of the ego.

Love of your soul and spirit, including full acceptance of any imperfections in your physical body, is empowering and freeing. The wisdom of Confucius tells us, 'If you look into your own heart, and you find nothing wrong there, what is there to worry about? What is there to fear?'

When you embrace the beauty of the soul within you, any physical impairment you may have will diminish in its significance. The more you can show compassion to your whole and complete self, the faster you will steer your focus away from your emotional discomfort or pain.

Please note—a million likes on your Facebook page or fans on your social media profile will never be enough if you do not like and love yourself. You must learn to love yourself as you are and your world as it is and carry on each day showing love and kindness to yourself, the world around you, and those you share your life with. Living your life from a place of compassion, kindness, faith, and love (rather than from a place of fear, blame, dislike, or hate) will transform you and make your world a much more joyful place.

DON'T KNOW WHERE TO START? HERE ARE SOME SIMPLE WAYS.

➢ **Be Someone Who Loves:** If you are struggling with the idea of loving yourself, begin by adjusting your mind and body to experience positive emotions by finding as many things to love and appreciate as possible. Notice more of what you love about the people you meet or who you spend time with. Notice more of what you love to experience or do or the things you love to have, hear, taste, touch, smell, or see.

➢ **Practise Self-Compassion:** Honour and respect your vulnerability. You are not a body that has a soul; you are a soul that is having a human experience. Acknowledge it is okay for you to make mistakes, struggle to lose or put on weight, or experience ups and downs with your moods and emotions. Understand that you do not need to be good at everything or have a physical body that seems to be as fit or active as others'. It is okay not to be as knowledgeable or skilled as a colleague, family member, friend, acquaintance, or neighbour. Practise compassion for yourself by accepting any shortcomings you may have just as much as your positive attributes, strengths, and passions. A great way to kickstart loving yourself is by consciously and consistently choosing to put your own compassionate and loving arms around *you*.

➢ *See Yourself as Worthy:* You are worthy of living a good life, and you deserve to be happy. Start respecting yourself by feeling deserving of spending time to take care of your desires and needs. Allow yourself to live your life filled up. Take time to nourish and care for yourself at a holistic level. Forgive yourself for ever thinking that you were not worthy or good enough.

➢ *Remain Aware of Your Inner Dialogue and Behaviour:* In those moments you find yourself struggling to love yourself, ask yourself how someone who loves you deeply would act towards you. What would they say to you? What would they do? How would they behave towards you? It is unlikely they would be unkind to you, criticize, or judge you. It is more likely that they would act lovingly towards you and speak words of compassion and kindness. Learn to be loving and forgiving to yourself, no matter your mistakes, shortcomings, challenges, or circumstances. Regularly ask yourself how someone who loves you deeply would act towards you and start acting towards yourself in that way.

➢ *Surround Yourself with People Who Feel Like Sunshine:* Jim Rohn tells us, 'You are the average of the five people you spend the most time with.' It makes sense, then, to remove yourself as much as possible from toxic relationships and choose to spend as much time as possible in the company of people who light you up, lift and nourish you, and inspire and motivate you.

Surround yourself with people who love and encourage you. Make a conscious choice to spend time with those who feel like sunshine and that you love to be around.

➤ *Be Persistent, Be Patient:* Self-love is something that needs to be practised daily and can take time to master. So be patient with yourself. Support yourself unconditionally through your hardest times and challenges. Do not let an odd day of hating yourself or of disliking your life get in the way of the bigger-picture better way of living, of you showing yourself care and compassion and being deserving of *you* giving love to *you*.

Keeping Things Simple: You must learn to love yourself wholly and without limits or conditions. When you love yourself fully, you will find you only want the best for yourself and are more likely to give yourself the best physical, emotional, and spiritual care. You are more likely to maintain new ways of thinking and being. Stepping up to take your unique place in this world will be easier when you respect yourself. Likewise, as you show self-love by honouring your happiness, desires, and needs, you will find the strength to commit to take actions that move you towards fulfilling your dreams.

RISE: CHOOSE TO LOVE

*Loving yourself starts with liking yourself, which
starts with respecting yourself, which starts with
thinking of yourself in a positive way.*

—Jerry Corstens

Your Day 23 *Rise* assignment is to spend the next few minutes
looking at yourself in the mirror through the eyes of someone
who dearly and unconditionally loves you. In the space below,
capture your insights about who and what you now see.

. . . .

. . . .

. . . .

. . . .

. . . .

. . . .

. . . .

. . . .

. . . .

. . . .

. . . .

. . . .

. . . .

DAY 24
UNLEASH YOUR POWER

We do not need magic to change the world; we carry all the power we need inside ourselves already: we have the power to imagine better.

—J.K. Rowling

Power

1. strength

2. the ability or capacity to do something or act in a particular way

3. the capacity or ability to direct or influence the behaviour of others or the course of events

—Definitions sourced from 1) Cambridge Dictionary, 2) Lexico Dictionaries, and 3) Lexico Dictionaries.

In a Nutshell: Power is the capability of doing or accomplishing something or acting in a specific way.

UNLEASH YOUR POWER

I t is time now to unleash your power. It is time to set free that inner strength that does not depend on outward things and can direct or influence not only the way you see yourself but what you do, who you become, how you see the world around you, and how willingly and enthusiastically you embrace your unique role whilst you are here on planet Earth. A big part of that power lies in the words you use—whether those words are spoken aloud or sung, said silently in your head, typed on your computer, or handwritten onto the page.

Today's module is empowering and impactful, so take your time to digest and implement what I share with you. The words you use have the power to either heal or harm you. They can make you feel better about yourself and help you own your place in the world—or they can act like restrictive chains around you and erode your soul and spirit and undo all the good work you have done up until now.

> THE WORDS YOU USE HAVE THE POWER TO EITHER HEAL OR HARM YOU.

Let me share private extracts from one of my journals (dated January 2003). Adjusting and reframing the words I used concerning myself and my perceived abilities freed me to move forwards and craft much change in my life. As you read the following journal extracts, I encourage you to pause from time to time and reflect on how the words I use may or may not relate to you.

Extracts from My Personal Journal January 2003
Maureen: Silencing My Inner Critic

My Thoughts: not good enough, fear of failure, fear of judgment, fear of what others think or say, not worthy of love, not liked, not enough energy, disabled, a lifetime of ill health and pain . . .

- ~~I am not good enough.~~ I am enough.

- ~~Fear of failure.~~ I can do this.

- ~~Fear of others' judgment.~~ I am the master of my mind, and it is what I think and believe that counts.

- ~~Fear of what others say.~~ I believe and trust in my voice. It is my opinion of me that is important.

- ~~People do not like me.~~ I like and love me.

- ~~I am not worthy of a great life.~~ I deserve to be happy and have success. I deserve to live my best life.

- ~~Life is hard for me. Life is restricted for me.~~ Life loves me, is good to me, and flows naturally through me.

- ~~I am disabled and limited in my ability.~~ When I expand what I think, I expand what I can do. When I expand what I do, I expand my world.

- ~~I have ongoing health issues.~~ My body and spirit have the power to heal.

My Feelings: fear, nerves, shyness, guilt, regret, lack of confidence, lack of self-belief, low self-esteem, self-conscious, feelings of weakness and vulnerability, feelings of not being good enough or worthy of love . . .

- ~~I am a disappointment.~~ My family is proud of me.

- ~~I lack confidence.~~ I have all the power, strength, and resources in me.

- ~~I feel physically weak and vulnerable.~~ I am mentally strong and powerful.

- ~~I feel forever exhausted.~~ I feel energised, nourished, and enriched.

- ~~I do not like myself. I do not feel good about myself.~~ I am a beautiful person. I feel love for me.

- ~~I feel anxious about my future.~~ I feel calm with a deep sense of knowing that all will be okay.

- ~~I feel guilty, for I am a burden.~~ My family loves me and wants only the best for me. They do things with love for me.

- ~~I feel weak and unable to look after myself.~~ A deep inner strength is within me, waiting to be unleashed.

ADJUSTING AND REFRAMING MY WORDS AND THOUGHTS

Time to Flip My 'But'

- ~~I want to go swimming, but I am very tired.~~ I am very tired, but I want to go swimming.

- ~~I would love to meet with friends, but my pain levels are high.~~ My pain levels are high, but I would love to meet with friends.

- ~~I want to go to the party, but I don't know how I will feel on the day.~~ I do not know how I will feel on the day, but I want to go to the party.

Time To Say 'Up Until Now'

- ~~I have been too tired.~~ *Up until now*, I have been too tired.

- ~~I feel uptight and anxious.~~ *Up until now*, I have been feeling uptight and anxious.

- ~~I have had no energy.~~ *Up until now*, I have had no energy.

- ~~I have not looked after myself very well.~~ *Up until now*, I have not looked after myself very well.

- ~~I am not good at taking rest when I need it.~~ *Up until now,* I have not been good at taking rest when I need it.

I feel raw and vulnerable sharing these journal extracts with you. However, it highlights how even the little things (e.g., changing the order of what goes before and after the word *but*) can be hugely impactful by sending a completely different message to your brain. Your mind sees the word *but* as negating what goes before it and therefore puts more focus and attention on the second part of the sentence. Try it for yourself and feel the difference it makes.

Similarly, the small difference of inserting the three short words *up until now* before a statement opens the doorway so that whatever you may have seen as being your factual reality can now perhaps be replaced by a different experience instead.

Most powerful is he who has himself in his own power.

—Seneca

BE CAUTIOUS

When adjusting or reframing the thoughts you hold about yourself, be careful of the language you use, for your mind does not pay attention to whether you do not want something or want something. You may think the two sentences below mean the same thing, but to the brain, they relay quite different messages. Try saying the following two sentences out loud, and you will feel and see what I mean.

- **I do not want to feel stressed.** (The brain homes in on the word *stressed* so it can make sense of what you are referring to—and it only brings you thoughts and feelings of stress.)

- **I want to feel relaxed.** (To understand the context of the sentence, the brain homes in on the word *relaxed* and brings you thoughts and feelings of relaxation.)

Notice how your brain picks the focus word of your sentence to make sense of what you mean.

Keeping Things Simple: Rather than thinking or stating what you do not want to have, be, feel, or achieve, flip your attention to what you do want instead. As you put yourself into a more positive state of mind and start to feel better about yourself and your life, your brain will automatically start looking for ways to help you achieve what you want.

RISE: UNLEASH YOUR POWER

Words can inspire, and words can destroy. Choose yours well.

—Robin Sharma

If you have had enough of feeling like a soul bound by chains in a chronically ill body, then you must stop seeing yourself and talking about yourself in a way that reaffirms or fortifies that way of thinking. Thus, your Day 24 assignment is in the form of a word swap challenge: do not mention the word *pain* for the next twenty-four hours.

You may choose to give it a more friendly, gentle, or comforting identity or name, but even better, turn all your focus on bringing greater feelings of comfort to yourself by avoiding talking about it at all.

As you move forwards, I encourage you to keep this word swap challenge going by consciously choosing not to name the discomfort you are feeling as 'pain' unless you are at a doctor or hospital appointment and doing so proves necessary.

Remember your words have power. Talking about what you are experiencing in your physical body as 'pain' only serves to reinforce the powerful negative connotations that your brain associates with that word.

DAY 25
ALLOW GOOD IN ABUNDANCE

Like the air you breathe, abundance in all things is available to you. Your life will simply be as good as you allow it to be.

—Abraham Hicks

Allow

1. to fail to restrain or prevent

2. allow the presence of or allow (an activity) without opposing or prohibiting

3. to make it possible for something to be done or to happen

—Definitions sourced from 1) Merriam-Webster,
2) Vocabulary.com, and
3) Cambridge Dictionary.

In a Nutshell: To allow is to permit something to happen or exist.

When you allow your circumstances to tear you down, it's unlikely that you will grow through them. Fate or a miracle cure don't determine whether challenges make you a better person or a bitter person— you do. The quality of life you experience within your unique set of circumstances ultimately comes down to you and what you allow yourself to focus on and believe.

THE QUALITY OF LIFE YOU EXPERIENCE WITHIN YOUR UNIQUE SET OF CIRCUMSTANCES ULTIMATELY COMES DOWN TO YOU AND WHAT YOU ALLOW YOURSELF TO FOCUS ON AND BELIEVE.

None of us like to think that we have played a part in adding to the difficulties and darkness we see. We assume our negative thoughts or feelings could not be of our own doing, but we all have a choice as to where we put our focus.

We can allow ourselves to focus on the good or bad, the happy or sad, the joyous and rewarding, or the soul-destroying and the painful. We can focus on our discomfort, or we can train our eyes and minds to see the good in life—and do all we can to live in a way that brings *more* good into our lives.

Be aware of the energy you give out to the world and the energy you allow to enter your personal space because what you allow perpetuates. Constant distractions and ongoing pain make it easy to become hacked by life. Once you've been drawn into the darkness, the tendency may be to settle there, despite the discomfort. That's why it's important to intentionally allow yourself to experience the good in life and to put your attention on abundance.

Put simply, life is a reflection of what you allow yourself to see.

What you allow is what will continue.

—Author Unknown

THE SECRET

I urge you to allow *change* to take a valued role in your life. Consciously allow in what you desire or want. Choose to let good thoughts and feelings and positive experiences enter, and at the same time, refuse to settle for less than your soul deserves.

Be brave and allow in peace.

Allow in comfort.

Allow in courage, strength, and mental resilience.

Allow in compassion and kindness.

Allow in understanding and self-worth.

Allow your support network to help and encourage you.

Allow in your Supreme Creator's presence.

Allow in the sunlight.

Allow yourself to see the beauty of nature.

Allow in the laughter of children.

Allow in gratitude and appreciation for life.

Allow in unconditional love for both yourself and others.

Trust and allow your soul to guide you to an oasis of calm and a feeling of home deep within you. Free your spirit to rise and your passion and enthusiasm for life to be reignited, refuelled, and rebirthed.

Keeping Things Simple: In life, whatever you keep the way open for and permit to enter will dictate the quality of both your today and tomorrow. Like the air you breathe, abundance in all things is still available to you. Do not lose sight of that. Refuse to allow pain and illness starve your soul of life.

RISE: ALLOW GOOD IN ABUNDANCE

*Like wildflowers, you must allow yourself to grow in
all the places people thought you never would.*

—E.V. Rogina

Your Day 25 assignment is to ask yourself the following
questions and jot down your answers in your journal. Answer
these questions every evening for the next week, then look
back over your entries and notice how much good you have
allowed to enter your life.

EVENING REFLECTION QUESTIONS

Did I allow myself to love today?

Did I allow myself to laugh today?

Did I allow myself to live today fully?

Did I allow myself to feel alive today?

Did I steer and allow my thoughts to focus on the good in life?

What one thing stands out as being the best thing about today?

What could I allow myself to do tomorrow to help me make
even more of a positive difference in my life?

PART FIVE

RISE

Shoot for the moon. Even if you miss,
you'll land among the stars.

—Les Brown

DAY 26
BE THE LIGHT

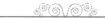

*Let your light shine so brightly that others
can see their way out of the dark.*

—Author Unknown

Light

1. radiant energy

2. something that makes things visible or affords
   illumination

3. An expression in somebody's eyes that shows what
   they are thinking or feeling

> —Definitions sourced from 1) Dictionary.com,
> 2) Dictionary.com, and
> 3) Oxford Learner's Dictionaries.

**In a Nutshell: Light is the brightness that makes it possible
to see things.**

As you begin to step into your power, you may find that others around you (including your family and friends) appear uncomfortable with the changes in your mindset and behaviour. *Do not let this hold you back!*

Not everyone will understand you or get you. Some people may be sceptical that your illness has ever been as severe as they thought it was. They may suspect you have been exaggerating the severity of your pain, or alternatively, they may fear your more positive persona will be short lived, that you are setting yourself up for a fall, or that your ego has got the better of you. Do not dim your light to appease them. There is no need to try to explain the changes within you. If you are constantly trying to justify your actions or prove your worth to others, you have already forgotten your value. Let the light you emanate do the talking for you.

When your loved ones and friends witness the sparkle in your eyes as you become more alive, they will be curious. You may even inspire them to seek positive changes for themselves.

Shine like the whole universe is yours.

—Rumi

CONNECT WITH YOUR SOUL MORE THAN YOUR PAIN

Your physical body may be labelled 'disabled' by society or doctors, but there is no need to be disabled in soul and spirit. Intentionally connect with your soul *more* than you connect with your pain. Reach inside you, ignite your light, and shine forth from within. Be willing to shine your light liberally; let it be of service to others. As you emanate a sense of oneness with the world despite the challenges you face, you will break down the barriers that have kept you from living fully alive and from releasing the healing power and passion of your spirit.

As you cast light on all things, you will drive out darkness. As your inner light grows, everything will begin to feel possible for you. From this sense of possibility, you will come to understand that healing is not all about curing. When you let go of the fight and struggle and allow peace to grow within yourself and in the world around you, you will illuminate a room merely by your presence.

> YOUR LIGHT IS OF SOUL AND SPIRIT. YOU ARE NOT MERELY FLESH.

Your light is of soul and spirit.

You are not merely flesh.

EMANATING THE LIGHT FROM WITHIN

We all have the light we need, we just need to put it into practice.

—Albert Pike

Everything you do in life is infused with the energy you bring to the task. If you want to become the most vibrant version of the light that is *you*, the following powerful visualisation will help. Make this exercise one of your non-negotiable nourishing daily practices. Take your time with it. The more you do the following visualisation, the more natural it will feel to step into that place.

Get as comfortable as you can, and still yourself by focusing on your breath. Breathe in (through your nose), and imagine a vibrant white or golden light entering, and as you breathe out (through your mouth), envisage all your inner staleness and darkness going away.

With each breath in and out, notice how much more alive you feel.

Now see in your mind's eye a more charismatic and confident you standing or sitting in front of you. Then imagine stepping or floating into that more alive and charismatic version of yourself.

See through their eyes, hear through their ears, and feel the feelings of being your more alive and vibrant self.

Now imagine that right in front of you is an even more animated and charismatic you—sitting or standing a little taller, emanating even more confidence and self-belief. Imagine stepping or floating into your even greater enlivened charismatic self.

See through their eyes, hear through their ears, and feel the feelings of your even more alive and brighter charismatic self.

Now notice that in front of you is an incredibly vibrantly alive *you*, with more passion and strength, more ease and natural comfort. Notice everything about you: how you are breathing, how you are standing or sitting, how you are holding and using your body, the expression on your face, how you are talking, how your voice sounds, the brightness of the shining light that emanates from you.

When you are ready, step or float into your even more enlivened charismatic self.

See through their eyes, hear through their ears, and feel the charisma and light pouring forth from within you.

Keep repeating the process, stepping or floating into a more and more animated, vibrant and alive you until you feel the light from within you shining outwards from every pore of your body.

Now imagine moving forwards into your day, using this inner light to face all your challenges and fears as this highest version of yourself.

Keeping Things Simple: An unlit candle does not shine. Once a candle is lit, however, it can be used to light another candle. In that moment of sharing its flame, the strength of the candle's light increases. You and I can shine and share light in the same way. We have the power to ignite the light within ourselves and reflect that light outwardly to ignite the souls of others because of the challenges and fire we ourselves have been walking through.

RISE: BE THE LIGHT

*A Warrior of the Light shares with others
what he knows of the path.*

—Paulo Coelho

Today, your *Rise* assignment is to spend the next few minutes thinking about the wisdom you have gained from living with pain and illness.

Below, jot down all the ways that you could help or guide others through their darkness by boldly shining your light and freely sharing what you have come to know.

. . . .

. . . .

. . . .

. . . .

. . . .

. . . .

. . . .

. . . .

. . . .

. . . .

. . . .

DAY 27
BE AT PEACE

*Be at peace with your own soul, then heaven
and earth will be at peace with you.*

—Isaac of Nineveh

Peace

1. freedom from disquieting or oppressive thoughts or emotions

2. calmness and tranquillity, a time when there are no wars going on or the state of having no war or conflict

3. a stress-free state of security and calmness . . . everything coexisting in perfect harmony and freedom

—Definitions sourced from 1) Merriam-Webster,
2) YourDictionary, and
3) Vocabulary.com.

***In a Nutshell: Peace is a calmness arising within you, saying,
'Rest easy, all is well'.***

My beautiful Gordon Setter support dog, Floyd, was my faithful companion and friend for eight years. Sadly, he was diagnosed with multiple tumours on both lungs, throughout his chest cavity, and on his bladder. A few days later, he made his journey to Rainbow Bridge.

In the wake of his death, I couldn't stop the tears from rolling down my cheeks. The devastating loss sucked the life right out of me. For the past eight years, Floyd stayed faithfully by my side. While I have been writing this book, he served as my chief cheerleader. Even now, I can imagine him in his usual daytime place—stretched out under my office desk with one paw across my ankle and his head resting on my feet.

I do not doubt that you will be familiar with the experience of death and the overwhelming feelings of sadness it brings. Death is a natural process and not something any of us can be freed from. In addition to Floyd, I have lost several precious family members, babies whilst still in my womb, close friends, work colleagues, and other beloved animal companions. Every one of those souls has touched my own deeply and will always have an incredibly special place in my heart. None of us is a permanent resident of this world; the life-death cycle is nature's way.

I had to recognise that I am only an
expression and symbol of the soul.

—Carl Jung

DEATH IS A NATURAL PROCESS AND NOT TO BE FEARED

The physical act of death is as natural as birth itself. Yet, because we worry about upsetting people and others worry that talking about death would make us feel uncomfortable, we often avoid the subject altogether. But death is not something to fear.

The truth is that although death is an end, it is also a beginning—a soul flowing seamlessly from having a physical experience to returning to the Universe or spirit world from whence it came.

Rest easy, and rest in peace. Death is not the finite end for any of us. It has never been, and never will be. I have had too many visits from my father and signs that he is forever around me since he died in 1991 to have any doubt. Perhaps I will share personal experiences from beyond the veil on another day or in another book.

In the meantime, all I ask is that you remain open to the idea that life will go on for you in a different format, with a different role to play, different things to do, different ways to be. I ask that you remain open to the idea that your soul and spirit will evolve further enriched from all the earthly lessons, learnings, and wisdom you have gained.

As your body comes to the end of its useful life on earth, your soul will rise from within to take its homeward flight.

DO NOT CLIP YOUR WINGS PREMATURELY

You are here with me now, and that means your heart is still beating. There is no need to let pain or illness dampen your soul and spirit or clip your wings prematurely. You have woken up this morning—and this means you are still meant to be here. You have much living left to do.

> YOU HAVE WOKEN UP THIS MORNING—AND THIS MEANS YOU ARE STILL MEANT TO BE HERE. YOU HAVE MUCH LIVING LEFT TO DO.

Every experience presents another opportunity to strengthen your wings so that you may rise like a golden eagle to serve others, shine your light, and encourage all whose lives you touch whilst you are here on earth to rise and do the same.

Replace your fear with faith, your turmoil with trust, any resistance with peace and grace. As a soul having an earthly journey in physical form, see how beautiful it truly is that you exist.

BE AT PEACE

If your physical illness has been deemed life-limiting or is progressively debilitating, it may be that you have already had personal thoughts or conversations about death with your loved ones or medical professionals.

Know you have a right to die well and with dignity just as you have a right to live well.

Do not be frightened to talk through with your loved ones how they can help you make your experience of death as meaningful a transition as possible when your time comes.

Rest easy. Be at peace with your soul. Live your life well, and do not let any ongoing pain or illness dampen your enthusiasm for life.

If it turns out that you are not on earth as long as some others, know it is because you are one of God's special messengers here to teach others the power of love, the truth of impermanence, the preciousness of life itself, and the importance of making the most of every heartbeat.

The death of my gorgeous boy Floyd reminded me of those truths once again. I feel privileged and blessed for the gift Floyd gave me as my amazingly loyal and faithful companion. His unconditional love uplifted me and supported me on good days and bad.

Whatever physical form we take, we are all souls on a journey. When our time on earth ends, perhaps we will rest awhile. As we look down on the loved ones we have left behind, may the light of our souls continue to support and guide them and offer comfort in their darkest moments.

Keeping Things Simple: Death happens to all of us. But it is not the end. You owe it to yourself to make the most of your life on earth whilst you are here.

RISE: BE AT PEACE

*There is no greater disability in society than
the inability to see a person as more.*

—Robert M. Hensel

It is Day 27, and your assignment today is to sit in quiet reflection. Allow your thoughts to be with your loved ones who have passed before you and explore what place they hold in your heart and how you mostly remember them.

Use the space below to freely jot down moments or situations when you feel you may have sensed their presence around you. Record the small events or happenings that have made you stop and think about them with the sense that, in spirit, they are still very much here.

. . . .
. . . .
. . . .
. . . .
. . . .
. . . .
. . . .
. . . .
. . . .
. . . .
. . . .

Day 28
PAY ATTENTION

Pay attention to the things you are naturally drawn to. They are often connected to your path, passion, and purpose in life. Have the courage to follow them.

—Ruben Chavez

Pay Attention

1. to be attentive to, become aware of, or be responsive (to someone or something)

2. the act of directing the mind to listen, see, or understand; notice

3. the regarding of someone or something as interesting or important

—Definitions sourced from 1) *Farlex Dictionary of Idioms*, 2) Cambridge Dictionary, and 3) Lexico Dictionaries.

In a Nutshell: To pay attention is to be aware of and attentive to someone or something.

I am certain that, as you have gone through life, you have felt a pull to go down a particular path, to take a certain course of action, or to be brave and make a specific choice—even if you do not know *how* you are going to make or achieve it. You may have a dream that keeps niggling away at you, nudging you to do something about it. Chances are, if you have not acted on it already, you have allowed your dream to be hacked; you have allowed yourself to be distracted and have focused your attention elsewhere. It may be that you felt you lacked the knowledge, experience, financial resources, ability, or courage to do the thing your heart was calling you to do.

If these desires and dreams are important to you, it is highly unlikely they will go away, for they come from a sacred place deeply rooted within you. If you fail to pay attention to them, their whispers will become louder, and at some point, start to scream.

When you dare to pay attention to your dreams and commit to doing all you can to achieve them, that same divine source that fired the dream within you will arise. It will deliver opportunities to help you with what you need to experience or know so you can move the dreams from concept to reality.

It is up to you to *pay attention,* however, to what the Universe is saying! Otherwise, you will miss out on the magic and mystery or possibility. Once you get clear on what you want and focus on playing your part to make it happen, a much bigger presence will step in to meet you.

The Brazilian writer Paulo Coelho summed it up so beautifully in his novel *The Zahir*: 'All you have to do is to pay attention; lessons always arrive when you are ready, and if you can read the signs, you will learn everything you need to know in order to take the next step.'

THE UNIVERSE HAS YOUR BACK

Your thoughts, feelings, words, and actions each produce energy which in turn attracts like energies. The Universe responds to the energy you emit by doing all it can to bring you what you most need in any given moment to help you (even if at times the experience would not be one of your choosing or is difficult or painful). The Universe will keep on sending you the same messages until you pay sufficient attention and listen. The whispers and nudges from the Universe will keep appearing, getting louder and more persistent; they will not go away until you notice and treat them as important and are willing to act on what your soul and spirit are calling you to do.

Here is the idea of what is called the law of attraction: Take action, and you'll be supported; there are no coincidences. The Universe will step in to help you; the Universe has your back.

Not convinced yet? Feeling sceptical? That is okay; I understand that. For a long time, I questioned it also. When Rhonda Byrne's book *The Secret* introduced me to the concept around twenty years ago, it all seemed too far detached from my reality at the time and way too simplistic. If life did work this way, I could not understand why we were not all taught about it by our parents or elders or at university or school. Also, the law of attraction didn't seem to apply to me. There was much pain and discomfort in my life, not to mention the poverty, pain, stress, and hate in the world. It did not seem to match up.

When I finally got my head around this way of thinking, however, I came to understand that in life that you are continually asking for what you want—or inadvertently asking for what you do not want—with the dominant vibration you emit. You cannot, for example, expect to attract a loving and caring relationship, a new job, or improved finances into your life if your dominant thoughts are of being no good at interviews, forever unlucky, and always in abusive relationships or debt. Likewise, you cannot expect to feel soul and spirit well if your dominant thoughts are of being depressed and ill and always stressed or anxious.

Positive change in your life requires you to start paying attention to that intuitive gut feeling that is your spirit and soul's way of calling you to attend to its needs. You must listen to what it is calling you to do, trust that voice within you enough to take inspired action, and with trust, belief, and focus, bravely and boldly take that next best step forwards on the path that feels most like home.

> POSITIVE CHANGE IN YOUR LIFE REQUIRES YOU TO START PAYING ATTENTION TO THAT INTUITIVE GUT FEELING THAT IS YOUR SPIRIT AND SOUL'S WAY OF CALLING YOU TO ATTEND TO ITS NEEDS.

Once you start acting on those intuitive nudges (no matter how small your steps may be), synchronicities and so-called 'coincidences' happen. You will find your attention drawn to certain events or circumstances or meeting or speaking with certain people. Nobel Prize winning author Doris Lessing said that coincidences are God's way of remaining anonymous. And very often, with hindsight, we can see that those coincidences brought us exactly where we needed to be and delivered the clear message we needed to see or hear to help bring our deepest desires to fruition.

Your deepest desires and heartfelt callings, however, will not come into your reality simply by putting them out to God in prayer. What *will* happen is that when the time is right and you are ready, the divine around and within you will draw your attention to the opportunities, circumstances, events, and people that are already here for you and in alignment with what you need.

A SPIRITUAL EXPERIENCE

That whisper you keep hearing is the universe trying to get your attention.

—Oprah Winfrey

Often, we deny spiritual experiences; we look instead for coincidences or reasons for them happening. We tell ourselves we have imagined them or dreamed them. We tell ourselves, 'That was weird!' or 'No way! That can't be!'

Spiritual experiences are, however, *spiritual* experiences. They may feel a little odd. We may feel self-conscious or even be slightly scared by them. Do not. There is no need to fear. Accept those moments, honour them, feel blessed by them. God is always talking to you and sending you little messages, reminding you to stop, look around, see and hear more, feel more, and listen. There is no need to understand the magic and mystery behind everything that happens in life. Accept whatever has happened. It was the way it was. It is what it is. Open your eyes, heart, mind, and soul; believe and know that these 'coincidences' are special moments. Feel love and gratitude for your soul and spirit being receptive to notice them, pay attention, and hear.

Keeping Things Simple: Pay attention to your intuitive nudges. They usually come from a heartfelt and sacred place.

RISE: PAY ATTENTION

The simple act of paying attention can take you a long way.

—Keanu Reeves

Your Day 28 assignment is to be more attentive to the dreams and desires trying to attract your attention. Perhaps you have a repeating thought or idea to go somewhere specific, meet up with someone, enquire about a new job or hobby, make an appointment with a particular specialist, paint or create something, pick up your guitar, tick an item off your bucket list, write to an old friend. Or maybe you are experiencing a growing feeling of a bigger presence supporting and guiding you, bringing certain people, opportunities, events, and happenings your way.

Simply allow your attention to go where it is naturally feeling drawn, and pay attention to what is calling you to see, hear, experience, do, or be. No matter how small a step you may take, take one inspired action *now* to acknowledge and explore that path.

DAY 29
RISE AND FLOW

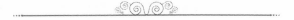

As you allow flow and change to occur, and as you keep looking inward, letting go of situations that cause you grief, and increasing the time spent in situations that allow you to be happy, your world will change.

—Doe Zantamata

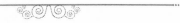

Flow

1. be abundantly present

2. to derive from a source

3. to move or run smoothly with unbroken continuity

> —Definitions sourced from 1) Vocabulary.com,
> 2) Merriam-Webster, and
> 3) American Heritage Dictionary.

In a Nutshell: Flow is a steady, fluid, and flexible movement progressing freely in a constant stream.

O n Day 28 I asked you to pay attention to the dreams and desires within you. Today our focus expands beyond the divine whispers and nudges to the messages being seeded in you by your mind, body, spirit, and soul. The purpose of paying full attention in a holistic way is to marry or meet the needs of your entire being and, in doing so, to establish the ability to rise and flourish.

Consider the following truths:

➤ *Truth #1:* Your body cannot do its best job if you do not give it the nourishment, fuel, exercise, and rest it needs.

➤ *Truth #2:* The mind cannot do its best job if you keep feeding it negative, self-critical remarks.

➤ *Truth #3:* Your soul cannot be fully unleashed and ignited if you keep fighting against things or putting resistance in the way to block it.

➤ *Truth #4:* Your spirit cannot rise and soar if you keep clipping its wings and encasing it like a bird in a locked cage.

When your life circumstances are interrupted and hacked by the presence of pain and illness, the difference between showing up to life half full or half empty becomes a choice that is only yours to make. Focusing on *being more* and experiencing more of the emotions you want to feel rather than aiming to *do more* to actively fight against what is real and present for you will cause a state of flow to arise with ease and grace from within you.

Flow means being fully immersed and involved in life—participating wholly and completely. Flow requires enthusiasm and passion for life and dancing with an energy and fluidity of movement between your head, heart, mind, body, spirit, and soul.

> *In a gentle way, you can shake the world.*
>
> —Mahatma Gandhi

Your Imagination and Intuition are Two of Your Greatest Gifts

Harnessing the power of your imagination (through seeing in your mind's eye and directing your attention to the outcome you want) and seamlessly blending it with the power of your intuition (to trust the choices and decisions that feel most like home to you) unleashes a powerful healing energy.

As you focus on *being more,* you will naturally find yourself wanting to *do more* without having to force anything or constantly drive hard with your foot on the accelerator pedal.

There is no downside to being in flow. As you find yourself doing more, you will begin to feel more rewarded, revitalized, alive, and awakened. Your soul and spirit will flourish within you. You will become less attached to your physical discomfort; your old patterns

> AS YOU FIND YOURSELF DOING MORE, YOU WILL BEGIN TO FEEL MORE REWARDED, REVITALIZED, ALIVE, AND AWAKENED.

of thinking or self-limiting beliefs; any lingering feelings of guilt, regret, or blame; and any fear of what other people may think or say. You will move into a state of connecting with the real *you* and experiencing a newfound strength, inner peace, and freedom.

Rather than always fighting for or against something, you will rise as a warrior of strength, courage, and mental resilience—of truth, wisdom, inner light, and grace.

You will find yourself moving from seeing a life of pain ahead to being excited by a life of passion and purpose. Rather than feeling alone in your struggles, you will feel supported. With trust and faith, you will have a deep-rooted knowledge that you have the power within you to deal with whatever life brings.

None of these things will have harsh self-restrictive boundaries to cross. When you get into a state of flow, you will remain in the joy of the moment without excuses or distraction. You will become the essence of your flow—confident in your abilities, moving from grieving for who you once were towards gratitude for who you are becoming. You will develop an ever-growing awareness of how precious and beautiful it is that you have been gifted this chance of life on earth and that you have a unique purpose to fulfil and a role to play.

You will feel alive and stay on task despite any ongoing physical discomfort. You will live your life not only as part of the Universe but with the Universe feeling part of you.

IT IS NOT ABOUT GOING WITH THE FLOW BUT BEING IN FLOW

The sun rises, and it sets. The tides of the river ebb and flow. Plants die back and rest in the cold dark of winter, then they turn their faces to the sun and burst back into life when the seasons change.

The key to living fully alive is to spend as much time in your 'heartspace' as you do in your headspace and free yourself to move with grace between them. The mountains and the valleys as well as the gently flowing rivers between them are all a natural part of your soul's journey. They are nothing to fear. On the contrary, they are all essential for your evolution and personal growth.

Wherever you go in life, show up filled up. Take your whole self, fully and completely. Rest in the knowledge that the human spirit is stronger than anything that could ever happen to it. Allow yourself to evolve and grow *within* the flow, *be* the flow, and embrace that both the darkness and the light of life are natural elements of the Universe and our Creator's way.

Keeping Things Simple: As you marry head and heart together, and allow flow and change to happen, your world becomes a better place.

RISE: RISE AND FLOW

And still I rise.

—Maya Angelou

Congratulations on getting this far! We are on the penultimate day of your elixir. It is Day 29, and your assignment today is to speak directly to your mind, body, spirit, and soul to gain clarity on what they most need so you can feel fully alive once more.

Do not speak about yourself in a head-thinking way, as in 'What do *I* want?' or 'What do *I* most need now?' Drop down and shift inward. Speak your words directly, first to your mind, then to your physical body, then to your spirit and your soul, asking, 'What do *you* most need from me? How can I help you? What do I need to do now, and who do I need to be now, to nourish, fuel, and help you best?'

Be attentive to what you intuitively hear, and jot down what becomes clear for you below.

. . . .

. . . .

. . . .

. . . .

. . . .

. . . .

. . . .

. . . .

. . . .
. . . .
. . . .
. . . .
. . . .
. . . .
. . . .
. . . .
. . . .
. . . .
. . . .
. . . .
. . . .
. . . .
. . . .
. . . .

DAY 30
SEIZE THE DAY!

Carpe Diem. Seize the day, boys. Make your life extraordinary.

—Tom Schulman, *Dead Poet's Society*

Seize the Day

1. to do the things one wants to do when there is the chance instead of waiting for a later time

2. make the most of the present moment

3. to make the most of today by achieving fulfilment in a philosophical or spiritual sense

—Definitions sourced from 1) Merriam-Webster,
2) Lexico Dictionaries, and
3) Wiktionary.

In a Nutshell: 'Seize the day' originates from the Latin phrase carpe diem, first used by the Roman poet Horace more than 2000 years ago, to mean you should enjoy life while you can.

On almost every memorial headstone you'll find the deceased's name, perhaps a few loving words, the date of the deceased's birth, and their death date. In the middle of those two dates is a dash. That dash may appear a small and insignificant horizontal line, yet as the symbol for a lifetime, it signifies so much more than any birth or death date or epitaph.

Every single heartbeat within you signifies *life,* and that same dash will appear on your memorial headstone when your time on earth comes to its conclusion. It is Day 30, the final day of your elixir, and it's time to fully embrace the significance of owning each heartbeat, living life fully, and making your time on this earth count!

> EVERY SINGLE HEARTBEAT WITHIN YOU SIGNIFIES LIFE.

The only way to make that dash between your birth and death date mean something is by embracing what it stands for and fully living it. Life is a doing word, an action, a decision, a participatory event. You can choose to be a bystander, sitting on the side-lines, and watch life happening for other people from a distance—or you can put yourself enthusiastically into life and show up wholly and completely: mind, body, heart, spirit, soul.

With the power of soul, anything is possible.

—Jimi Hendrix

FOCUS ON ACTION, NOT EXCUSES

There is *always* something you can do to improve your situation and enhance or transform your experience of your world.

If you cannot run a marathon, you can choose to support a friend who can. If you cannot go hillwalking, perhaps you can still go and sit at the side of a lake or loch, breathe in the fresh air, listen to the birdsong, and appreciate nature's beauty.

If there is a dream within you—something you want to achieve in your lifetime, or somewhere you want to go—focus on *how* to make what you may have deemed too difficult or impossible happen.

It is okay to have a bad day, shed tears, get angry, and feel sorry for yourself. All these emotions are a natural element of being human. If you are serious about living your best life, however, you must allow yourself to feel what you feel and then consciously turn your soul to the sun, pick yourself up, and remind yourself that you can and will get through it. Tomorrow is another day to start afresh—another twenty-four hours and another precious 100,000 heartbeats.

Some people have experienced the most horrendous things and found a way to navigate to their passion and joy in life again. The Mexican artist Frida Kahlo was only six years old when polio left her paralysed. The virus caused severe damage to her legs, but her disability did not stop her from becoming world famous. Her inspiring words, 'Feet what do I need them for / If I have wings to fly[?]'[11] are a great reminder that every single heartbeat presents us with a fresh opportunity to rise and flow from the darkness and seize the day.

When you wake up tomorrow, know that not everyone will have that same privilege. The finite number of heartbeats will expire for some people, and they will leave this world behind. I make no apology for bringing this harsh reality to your attention—every single day on earth you have from now on is one less day you will have left to live.

EMBODY ENTHUSIASM, NOT DEFEAT

With the reality in mind that time on earth is finite, I urge you to stop focusing on your illness or suffering and consciously choose to focus on *doing* not dreaming, *thriving* not surviving, *fully living* rather than existing.

> ➤ Pop singer Lady Gaga is one of the most famous artists in the world and sells millions of copies of her albums despite living with the painful and debilitating chronic condition of fibromyalgia.

> ➤ Stephen Hawking left an outstanding legacy as a great scientist despite having motor neurone disease, which saw him paralysed from head to toe for over thirty years and having to use a voice synthesiser to communicate.

> ➤ Despite being born without arms and legs, Nick Vujicic is a dynamic young evangelist who travels the world changing lives.

You achieve wonderful things when you choose to put yourself wholly into life. Sharing the inspiration of Rumi,

'There is a morning inside you waiting to burst open into Light.'[12]

Congratulations!

It is the final day of your elixir.

Be proud of how far you have come.

It is time for you to start shining your light and making every heartbeat count.

Keeping Things Simple: How fully you choose to live and embrace life comes down to you.

RISE: SEIZE THE DAY!

The living soul of man, once conscious
of its power, cannot be quelled.

—Horace Mann

The final *Rise* assignment of your 30-Day elixir is to go to YouTube. Search for '"Creating the Spectacle!" Online - Part 1 - Finding Freedom'[13] and watch the incredible video of a lady called Sue Austin fulfilling her dream of scuba diving in a wheelchair. I was first introduced to this video in Kary Oberbrunner's *Wall Street Journal* and *USA Today* best-seller *Unhackable* (upon which this book is based). Mesmerized, I saved the link to my computer to watch it again and again.

Do yourself a favour now. Gift yourself the next five minutes to be inspired by this amazing lady. If there were ever a way of encouraging you to make the most of your 'dash' and make the very most of your time on planet Earth, *this is it.*

AFTERWORD:
UP CLOSE AND PERSONAL

If you have not yet received the miracle you've been praying for, the best thing to do is become a miracle for someone else!
—Nick Vujicic

You Are Enough
ACCEPTANCE OF THAT IS EMPOWERING

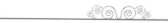

Acceptance doesn't mean resignation; it means understanding that something is what it is and that there's got to be a way through it.

—Michael J. Fox

I hope that what I have shared with you in *Unhackable Soul* has reignited a spark of fire in your soul and inspired you to think anew about your life and the unique role you play whilst on this earth.

I have never promised that this book would bring you a physical cure or magic fix. There is no one-size-fits-all answer for any of us. In truth, some days, I struggle to hobble even a few short steps, and it is almost impossible to get my shoes on. As I wrote these words, my feet were heavily swollen and discoloured and felt as if they were fire. Around each of my ankles, it seemed as though I wore a red-hot barbed wire tourniquet. The tendons in my legs felt so tight, like elastic bands stretched to their maximum capacity, that at any moment they might have snapped.

Every day, my bones hurt. My atrophied muscles throb. The fiery nerve pain, never-ending biting and stinging wasps and ants, and burning pins and needles ferociously radiate from the tips of my toes all the way up both legs to my buttocks and bladder in a bid to flee the internal burning lava. My legs and feet spasm with such violence that it is hard to breathe.

My hands, arms, and shoulders are purple and swollen. They feel as if they are being ripped from my body as I write this. I hear the blood flow in my head loudly pounding and rhythmically whooshing. My clear soup lunch stayed down all of twenty minutes before my stomach decided to reject its contents yet again.

Suffice it to say, my illness is complex and widespread. It would be easy to let my pain consume me and take my mind to a dark place. The amazing thing is that whilst everything that is happening to my physical body appears, at an external level, scary, I do not *feel* scared at all. It is as it is for me; I am where I am. And I know I can handle it, whatever *it* is.

Through the years, I have realised there is no need to give brain space to thoughts of a bleak future or envisage a tortuous lifelong sentence. There is also no need for me to constantly fight against something over which I do not have full control. Life goes on for me as it does for you. I can still thrive despite my circumstances. I can flourish. I can embrace the preciousness of each day as it unfolds before me and deal with each situation as it arises to the best of my ability.

I am not obliged to follow a predetermined, set-in-stone journey. Acceptance of my situation as it is right here, right now, acts only as a truthful starting point for my deeper personal growth and the conscious making of more meaningful decisions as I move forward.

This is a complete contrast from the way it used to be for me. I fought the acceptance of my situation for years.

When doctors initially told me that an incurable, progressive neurological illness was a real possibility for me—and later, when doctors confirmed it—the prognosis rocked me to the core. I abhorred the idea. A life of being disabled in a wheelchair, assisted by carers, and consumed by severe, relentless pain was not something I had planned for or envisaged. I could not help thinking this was not how my life was meant to be.

I did my best to block it out of my mind and carry on as normal. Putting up a barrier to the word *acceptance,* I fought it with every fibre of my being. I was forever trying to run in the opposite direction, away from the picture of a life I did not desire.

FIGHTING THE FIGHT AND RESISTING

At the outset of this book, I told you about the dark November morning in 2002 when the truth of my reality hit home for me. I found myself responding to my situation in the only way I knew how at that time—by fighting against it even harder. In the years that followed, I set physical goals and embarked on hours upon hours of physiotherapy and hydrotherapy. I followed restrictive diets, used empowering mantras, practised positive visualisation, and made many lifestyle changes to eliminate unhelpful stress from my life, including leaving a long-term unfulfilling marriage. Willingly, I embraced new medications and complementary therapies. I started trying anything and everything in the hope that I could craft a much brighter future than the one life had seemingly mapped out for me. I wanted to prove the medical profession wrong. I wanted to *fully live*.

Whilst my hard work over the next decade did eventually pay off, it felt as though I was in a constant battle; I was forever pedalling uphill against a gale-force wind. Rather than fighting *for* my burning desire for a brighter future, I had inadvertently become consumed in battling *against* a life I did not desire or want. It was hard. It was exhausting and physically and emotionally draining.

I got so caught up in the process of trying to be the stronger opponent against my illness that I lost sight of who I truly was and neglected to fully appreciate the life I had available to me in the present, *right here, right now.*

Did my fight and resistance to my illness bring rewards? Yes, in many ways, fighting against my illness brought positive and meaningful rewards for me. Through my mind-over-matter sheer guts and determination, against all odds, I successfully turned my life and health around. I felt like Superwoman; I had developed the courage and mindset of a champion. In truth, I started to believe I had this thing we call *life* sussed.

Wanting to put purpose to all I had learned and gone through, I trained as a life and mindset coach, studied neuro-linguistic programming (NLP) and hypnosis, and set up my successful coaching practice helping others who were going through challenging circumstances.

I even started to write a book about my ten-year 'power of the mind healing journey' and got the interest of a major publisher. In the book, I shared the steps I had taken to beat my illness and successfully transform my life.

It was only a matter of time, however, before I had to face my truth.

I started falling a lot and dropping things. My speech was slurred at times, and I would get blurred vision. I experienced much more intense nerve pain and burning, disabling muscle spasms, fatigue and brain fog, and balance issues that had me walking as if I were drunk. Nerve damage remaining from previous years continued to necessitate catheterising my bladder and irrigating my bowels through a permanent stoma daily.

Even so, I was exceptionally good at hiding my growing discomfort from others. I visited family, worked with clients on either side of my rest times, and never openly discussed my physical concerns. By not putting importance on my increasing pain, I was hoping that my challenges would miraculously ease into the background, not be visible to others, or go away.

I bought into my own story that I was fully cured and kept up outward pretences. I openly voiced that the power of my mind was my healing key.

A Bad Fall Intervened

A bad fall at the beginning of 2015 further complicated my internal battle. The fall severely compressed an artery and nerves in my shoulders, arms, and chest. In typical Maureen style, I did my best to block it out of my mind. I played it all down at first and outwardly kept the smile on my face. I said I was okay—but I wasn't. Complex diagnostic tests explored the problem and surgeries were planned. Without knowing how much of the nerve damage could be reversed or healed, I felt myself spiralling towards a black hole again as the feeling of fighting hard against a bleak future once more reared its ugly head.

My Head and Heart Pulled in Different Directions

My heart and gut were calling me to accept and acknowledge the challenges that my physical health presented, but my overthinking head told me that would be a sign of weakness and giving up. The result was that I lived the life of two different people for quite some time—my head and heart were completely out of alignment. I was doing all I could to portray the outer mask and persona of the resilient, fully happy and healthy ever-smiling mindset coach who had risen against the odds to prove that anything and everything is possible. All the while, my emerging spiritual soul called me to step into the reality of my ongoing physical health complexities and into the raw, vulnerable truth of me.

I was sitting in my kitchen writing in my private journal one morning in 2016, and with incredible ease and grace that I still find it hard to fathom, true acceptance of my situation fell into place for me. In that memorable moment, I felt the most overwhelming surge of soothing, awakening warmth and peace. Rather than opening the door onto a darkening path (to a future I had spent much of my life fighting), accepting my situation meant I found myself dropping beautifully and gently into perfect alignment with the real me.

What struck me most at the time was that nothing bad had suddenly happened; I was still exactly where I was, and nothing had physically changed for me. No doom and darkness had descended. The bleak future I had fought so hard against had not suddenly come into my reality. It was the opposite: I felt empowered and enlightened. I felt alive, secure, and safe.

And in a deep, heart-warming surge, the light came on for me, and my truth became clear:

I am not my physical body.

I am not my self-limiting mind.

I am the soul and spirit within.

I am me.

All pictures of a bleak future and fear of further ailing health simply dissolved for me in that very instant. A newfound sense of freedom, faith, and trust entered, and from that moment, they have never left. These days, a flowing, soothing calm runs

I AM NOT MY PHYSICAL BODY.
I AM NOT MY SELF-LIMITING MIND.
I AM THE SOUL AND SPIRIT WITHIN.
I AM ME.

through my core and allows me to differentiate between my current pain and circumstances and to see that any negative thoughts or images of suffering I chose to attach to it are optional. Acceptance of my truth and reality has led me to a place of deep peace, authenticity, courage, trust, and faith within me.

Seeing my truth as it is—free of judgement and with no need to determine whether it is fair or unfair, good, bad, or otherwise—enables me to live fully. I can breathe, think, and act from the exact truth of where I am. In my mind and soul, like the peaceful azure sea of Galilee, I enjoy a deep contentment and calmness that has found rest.

Fighting against your illness or doing your best to ignore or deny your pain and discomfort may feel as if it's the only or best solution to you for a while; however, it is not how you will find lasting peace within your situation, a newfound enthusiasm and zest for life, or healing. Fighting against something feels like fighting. Battling something feels like a battle. But rising from within your circumstances and in the direction of your heartfelt desires comes from the quiet acceptance of what is. It comes from freeing and unleashing your soul and spirit to live with purpose and enthusiasm for the life you have available right now.

Acceptance makes an incredible fertile
soil for the seeds of change.

—Steve Maraboli

ACCEPTANCE: THE TRUTH AND FACTS

➤ Acceptance does not necessarily mean liking, wanting, endorsing, choosing, or supporting something. You simply allow yourself to embrace the moment, including the aspects of your truth and reality that may be challenging or cannot be changed.

➤ Acceptance does not mean that you must stop trying to improve or change things or that your situation will necessarily be as it now is forever. On the contrary, acceptance brings freedom as you move forwards moment by moment to make more positive conscious decisions and take inspired action from a known starting place.

➤ Acceptance is not something to fight or fear—it opens the door to fresh ways of thinking and being and shines light on a more authentic life.

➤ Acceptance leads you to unfold an ever-deepening inner journey of increasing self-awareness, meaningful reflection, personal learning, soul and spirit growth, valuable gifts, insights, and freedom to be you.

➤ Your life choices can come from your thoughts, feelings, and actions that are birthed, grown, and nurtured in that new and empowering acceptance space.

Keeping Things Simple: Acceptance says, 'It is true. This is my situation and my reality at this present moment. I can now breathe, think, choose, live, and act from here. Within

the space of acceptance, I can open my arms and heart wide to make the most of my today, my tomorrow, and whatever my future brings.'

A PERSONAL MESSAGE

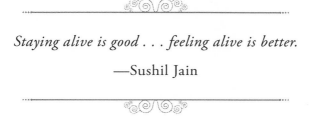

Staying alive is good . . . feeling alive is better.
—Sushil Jain

As you move forwards, be gentle and patient with yourself; sustainable change takes time and is unlikely to happen overnight. Healing takes time—no matter the shape or form your holistic recovery may birth. If you have been going through a difficult period recently, know that there will come a time when you feel better than this. I cannot promise you it will be today. Nor can I promise you it will be tomorrow. But believe and know that by taking one next best step at a time and following the fundamental principles I share with you in this book, that day *will* come.

So be kind to yourself, loving, and supportive. Keep on living until the day comes when you feel fully alive once more. There is no pleasure in allowing your pain and illness to dictate or rule your life—being physically alive and breathing but feeling dead on the inside.

We *all* fall at times, but we all can rise. We all make mistakes, but we all can learn from them. We all get knockbacks at times, but we all can pick ourselves back up from them. We all can move through personal hurt to evolve and heal.

As you move forward, consciously take ownership of the pictures you make in your head and the stories you tell yourself. Reassess the beliefs you hold, be attentive as to how you spend your days, and choose wisely the people you spend most of your time with. In addition, examine your relationships—with yourself, with others, with the Universe, with God—and develop those relationships in a way that supports and serves your well-being best.

Make this your time to turn the page and start a new chapter of your story. Choose to live with greater enthusiasm, joy, and passion, and deeper peace, meaning, and purpose. You and I are courageous souls on a similar journey. We owe it to ourselves to live *fully alive*, and despite our challenging circumstances to make a difference to the world whilst we are here on earth by shining our unique light and showing up filled up and being fully here.

Be proud. I believe in you.

LIVING WELL WITH PAIN AND ILLNESS

*The difference between a good life and a bad
life is how well you walk through the fire.*

—Carl Jung

Over the last three and a half decades, I have learned a lot about living with pain and illness. It's only fair to say it hasn't always been the smoothest of journeys. What I have come to know for certain, however, is that when it comes to living well with pain and illness, the following things really help:

BUILD A STRONG TEAM AROUND YOU.

Develop a supportive network of people around you who believe in you, your dreams, your hopes, and your abilities—and who will stand strong by you in your desire to embrace and live your life fully. Let them know how much you appreciate them and how much you value the part they play in your life.

BE YOUR OWN HEALTH ADVOCATE AND GURU.

See your physical and mental health as being your responsibility—not the responsibility of your doctor or any other health professional, family member, colleague, or friend. It is *your* body, mind, heart, soul, and spirit. Whilst it is important to be open to the knowledge, experience, and advice of health specialists, ultimately, it is up to you to educate yourself and best understand your health condition to look after yourself well.

STAY ON TOP OF CURRENT RESEARCH.

Keep researching treatment options and new developments regarding your specific health condition, sharing and discussing your findings with your doctors. Even if your doctors have told you there is no effective medication or cure for your health condition now, it does not necessarily mean there never will be.

SEE YOURSELF AS A WHOLE PERSON.

Treat yourself holistically: mind, body, spirit, soul. See that they are all elements of you and interconnected; you must treat yourself kindly and nourish and feed each of part of yourself well. Don't put all your focus and energies into one or two of them and starve or ignore the rest.

DEVELOP COMFORT AND COPING PRACTICES.

Be open-minded to trying things that may help you. Whether it is listening to music or watching a film to distract yourself from pain, visualisation, meditation, or mindfulness, pottering in the garden, going to a support group, taking a drive in the country, doing a little cooking, or picking up the phone to talk with a friend, the list is endless. Utilise the things that help you positively and beneficially and have the courage to minimise or park the rest.

EXPAND YOUR WORLD—DO NOT KEEP YOUR WORLD TOO SMALL.

Reach out to others and enjoy their company on the days you feel up to it; be productive and still go places and actively do things. Focus on doing what you *can* do—not on any limitations your illness imposes on you. Showing up filled up and participating as fully as you can in life will bring you more feel-good feelings than isolating yourself and retreating from life or withdrawing into your shell.

BE OPEN TO CONVENTIONAL MEDICAL PRACTICES AS WELL AS COMPLEMENTARY TREATMENTS AND THERAPIES.

You are an individual and unique. Therefore, remain open-minded regarding treatments and therapies that may help you. Accept that no one size fits all or is the perfect treatment that will work for everyone, but the options are plentiful. If something interests you or feels right to you and is unlikely to do you any harm, be willing to try it and trust that you know your body best.

TRUST YOUR VOICE (AND DO NOT BE AFRAID TO SPEAK UP)!

Doctors are not God; they are human and can have their off days like the rest of us. However, any doctor who is rude, arrogant, or condescending to you—dismissive, uncaring, judgmental, not understanding your condition and how it affects you, or accusing you of exaggerating your pain—is not the right doctor for you. You deserve the best care and treatment, including a doctor on your side who wants only the best for you. Be prepared and willing to change your GP if need be or change your practice until you find a doctor who fully supports you. Seek another opinion from a different consultant if need be. Trust your voice, speak up, and be heard.

BEFRIEND YOUR BODY; IT IS NOT YOUR ENEMY.

Work with your body, not against it. Your body is part of you and not the enemy. Take quiet time regularly to ask your body, 'How can I best serve you? How can I best help you? What do you most need from me today to help you experience greater comfort or function best?' Ask, listen, trust, and respond. Get to know your body well and confidently act on its needs.

FEEL IT. HEAL IT. LET IT GO.

Your body has enough to contend with without adding negative thoughts and emotions for it to deal with as well. Allow yourself to grieve if need be; feel angry; acknowledge regret, guilt, or blame; question 'why me?'; or spend a short while feeling sorry for yourself and in victim mode. *You are human, and it is natural to feel these emotions and work through these things.* Hanging on to negativity, however, does not help. A negative mind will never bring you a positive experience of life.

PAY LITTLE ATTENTION TO DISCOURAGEMENT.

See that a bad day is simply a bad day and does not necessarily need to turn into a bad week, bad month, or bad year for you. Reminding yourself that you only ever must deal with the moment you are in now can help you get through those more difficult days when darkness descends.

RESPECT AND PROTECT YOUR OWN SPACE.

Protect your space and establish your boundaries when it comes to the advice you may receive from well-wishers, for example, 'Have you tried XYZ yet?' 'My friend had that and says she's cured now.' 'Perhaps you should try some exercise or get out more?' Offer the benefit of the doubt to people and believe they have offered their advice with the best intentions. Listen and take on board any advice you feel may be helpful. Park the rest, however—and do not feel bad about it. You alone are the expert on your own life.

SPEND MORE TIME IN YOUR HEART, LESS TIME IN YOUR HEAD.

Avoid complicating life by overthinking every decision, action, communication, or thought. Keep things simple (and a lot less tiring and stressful) by thinking less and feeling more. Learn to trust your intuition: the essence, truth, soul, and heart of *you*.

BELIEVE AND KNOW YOU CAN HANDLE IT— WHATEVER 'IT' IS.

Worry is like a rocking chair. It will give you something to do, but it will not get you anywhere. Live with faith and trust. Believe and know that you have all the power within you to deal with whatever life brings. One moment, one next best step at a time, is all you ever need to focus on.

FIND YOUR PEOPLE; CONNECT WITH YOUR TRIBE.

When it comes to chronic pain and illness, unless someone else has 'got it', it is unlikely they will truly get you. Join an uplifting and positive support group where you can mix with others who clearly understand the pain and challenges you go through without the need for you to be constantly explaining your illness or talking about or focusing on the problems you have. Alternatively, find and work with an inspiring personal coach or mentor who has experienced similar things or walked the same path you are on.

ALWAYS REMEMBER LIFE IS PRECIOUS.

Whilst death may be the destination of your physical body (and you can rest at peace in the knowledge that your spirit and soul will live on), when you wake up in the morning and find you are still breathing, rise and give thanks. *Know that your job on earth is not yet done*!

MY DEEPEST DESIRE NOW

She made broken look beautiful and strong look invincible. She walked with the Universe on her shoulders and made it look like a pair of wings.

—Ariana Dancu

M y deepest desire as we get ready to part for now is that the insights, practices, and knowledge I have shared with you in this book act as a catalyst for you to think anew about your circumstances and that you embody them as you move forwards to help craft positive and meaningful change in your life. I encourage you to dive back into *Unhackable Soul* and your 30-day elixir often. Use this book as your supportive guide and companion rather than a fleeting visitor left on a shelf to gather dust.

There is a difference, however, between *knowing* the path and *taking* the path. There is a difference between gaining new ways of thinking and putting those new ways of thinking into actionable practice. If you want to craft change in your world, commit to *being* the change. Whilst pain and illness may continue to shape your overall journey, it need not define you now or ever. A strong positive mental attitude married with enthusiasm and joy for life will create more magic and miracles for you than any treatment or wonder drug. At any given moment, you have the choice to rewrite your story. You have the power to ignite and unleash the soul and spirit within you and say, 'A life defined or overshadowed by pain and illness is not how my story ends.'

TOGETHER WE CAN MAKE A DIFFERENCE

Throughout this book, our pain has united us. As we both move forwards now, it is important we know we *can* make a difference. By standing in grace and acceptance of our reality and truth and embracing an unconditional joy and love for life despite the often-difficult roller coaster ride we are on, we can gently yet boldly encourage a ripple of change in others towards a more understanding, more compassionate and tolerant, more real, more truthful, much less judgmental, and kinder world.

For life is not about finding ourselves. We are not lost, nor broken—we have never been. Life's journey is about discovering, honouring, and embracing the truth of who we were born to be.

OWN WHO YOU ARE

Please know there is no 'right' way to live with a chronic illness. Despite any advice you may be given along the way, there is only *your* way. You and I can only live our lives for ourselves. No one can do it for us or tell us what is right or wrong for us; we must honour who we truly are and choose to live the best way that we can.

Nobody is superior to you. Nobody is inferior. Each of us is unique and beautifully perfect in our imperfections. You are you. I am me. It is up to me to discover and embrace my Being. Likewise, it is up to you to find and welcome yours.

It may be that you haven't agreed with everything I have said in this book. You may not be at a similar stage in your illness or experiencing the same deep level of spiritual awareness. *I want you to know that is okay.* The world of chronic pain and illness is not an easy one to live in; it can make you doubt and question or be dismissive of all sorts of things.

In truth, we are all at different stages on our journeys, opening our gifts and lessons in our perfect timing. Wherever you are now, *you* be strong; your pain deserves its truest voice. Being fully alive does not mean only embracing the happy or good times in life. Being fully alive means shining forth a love for life itself and an open willingness to embrace it all.

I have put my pain to purpose by writing this book and sharing what I have learned about living with pain and illness. I have metabolized my pain as positive energy. If what I have shared with you in *Unhackable Soul* has inspired or resonated with you somehow, I invite you to reach out to me for further support. You can connect with me via my website at MaureenSharphouse.com where you can explore my mentoring and coaching programmes and access free personal development resources. You will also find links at the back of this book to connect with me on social media.

The bottom line is, I am here for you and would love to help you.

There is no need for you to navigate your pain and illness challenges alone.

READY TO HEAR THE GOOD NEWS?

Restoring fire and passion back into your spirit and soul and becoming fully alive and Unhackable has serious advantages. The difference in the quality of the life you live is transformational. Here are four of the most common benefits:

1. *Productivity*: As you become more enthusiastic about your daily life, you find yourself doing more.

2. *Fulfilment*: You feel more fulfilled and live your life with a greater sense of purpose.

3. *Clarity and Focus*: You become more focused and have greater clarity about what and who is important to you. As a result, you take action to achieve your heartfelt desires and dreams.

4. *Space and Freedom*: As you redirect your attention away from your pain and illness, you create more space and freedom in your life for other things, including rewarding relationships, greater contentment, a newfound zest for life, more success, and fun.

Keeping Things Simple: Reigniting the light within you, and keeping it burning brightly, is the perfect elixir for living your best life.

A PARTING STORY

Light the Dark

I will love the light for it shows me the way;
yet I will love the darkness for it shows me the stars.

—Og Mandino

Saturday, 27th January 2017, 10:35 pm

As I flick the light switch, instant darkness descends. A child-sized gasp for breath cuts through the now uncomfortable quiet, replacing what up until this moment has been a room of joyous laughter and giggling children's charm. The newfound silence finds us huddling together on the beige leather sofa, two adults and four children now closely conjoined in our glass-roofed central atrium.

Four of my precious grandchildren are on a sleepover at Granny's house, and we have had such a wonderful evening. We have laughed so much it was heart-warming and belly-aching—and when the rubbing of eyes and yawning made their appearance, the youngsters willingly got on their pyjamas and volunteered to go to bed. I invited them, however, to a late-night treat, telling them I had a special magic show I wanted them to see in the atrium.

But with the simple flick of the light switch that plunges us all into darkness, I sense I may have called the children's fun evening to an abrupt end. The unexpected darkness unnerves them big time. I do my best to reassure the children they are safe and ask them to trust me. I tell them there is something incredibly special I want them to see.

'I'm scared, Granny. It's so dark! I hate the dark. What if there is a monster?'

I feel an anxious grabbing of my arm and hand. Faith, the youngest, attempts to bury her head and face behind my shoulders. The darkness of the night turns even darker; a wave of a chill goes through the air.

'You are going to have to trust me on this. If you are brave enough to open your eyes in a moment and look into the dark, you will see something quite wonderful.'

'I'm scared, Granny. . . .'

'Let us all open our eyes together. What do you say? Have we a deal?'

I sense a nod of heads, one by one, accompanied by a gentle mumble of general agreement, each child both giving and taking comfort from their siblings' mounting bravery and trust.

'One, two, three, let's open our eyes.'

'I can't see anything, Granny! Just darkness!'

'Simply sit awhile—and trust me. And when you feel ready, look up at the glass ceiling. For I promise you, within the darkness, you will find real-life magic up there.'

It is inevitable. At first, as each child cracks open their eyelids, they see nothing. Then the cold shivery darkness consumes them; I can feel their growing pain. Lack of belief in seeing anything but the dark restrains them from seeing more.

Some gentle words of encouragement, however, start to lift their spirits. Although still anxious, they bravely begin to look steadily upwards towards the dark sky visible through the sloped glass ceiling. And as their fear subsides and their eyes adjust, the magic begins to happen: the stars appear.

At first, a solitary bright star shines like a diamond in the dark, making its regal royal entrance.

'I can see something, Granny! I can see a bright light! I can see a star shining up there!'

Then another star—and another. And another—and so the stars keep appearing.

Soon hundreds of stars make their proud appearance; the sky becomes ablaze with a divinely magical sparkling light show. Small eager voices, joy and laughter, and pointing fingers break through the stilled silence. And within a few moments, the experience of Granny's sleepover evening has come to life again and is transformed.

Never before have I seen so many stars at the same time shining so brightly. I put my trust in the Universe, and it has answered. It has delivered the magical experience I so wanted my grandchildren to see.

Nothing has changed for any of us at a material level: We are still sitting close together, huddled on the beige leather sofa. The room is still dark all around us. The sky above is the same jet-black colour as before.

But something profound has happened.

It is not the black of the darkness into which we are all now looking. Despite the darkness, and right there amid the darkness, we are all seeing and appreciating so much more.

Our focus has been drawn to the magical twinkling light show as it unfolds with grace before us. It is not that the stars have newly formed in this exact moment. On the contrary, they were there all along this evening and have been visible since sundown; it is only that we did not actively look for them or notice them before.

'Granny. That really is magic.'

'What do you mean, Caleb?' I ask, inviting some real-life thinking.

'Well, if we hadn't looked right into the darkness, we might not have seen the stars at all.'

The wise young guru had spoken. And within his wise words, there lies an important message:

Stars don't shine without darkness.

That sounds a lot like you and me.

Namaste, my dear reader. May the road rise to meet you as you continue your journey.

The light in me honours and respects the light that is in you.

Maureen

MAUREEN SHARPHOUSE
Live a life of no limits

My Manifesto

STOP expecting somebody or something else to come along and fix things for you.

Too often we feel trapped or stuck in our circumstances. Too often we sit and wait, and pray for the 'magic wand'. Too often we don't see that we have choices and options. Too often we settle for what feels second best.

 WHY?

We perceive limitations, closed doors and boundaries. We let fear of failure stop us. We let lack of courage keep us small. We silence our inner voice telling us there's more for us to do and be in life. We worry about judgment of others. We put importance on their voice.

WHAT IF YOU THREW OFF THE SHACKLES OF THE LIFE YOU'VE BEEN LIVING? WHAT IF YOU GAVE YOURSELF PERMISSION TO FULLY EXPRESS YOU?

IT'S YOUR LIFE your mind, your body, your choices It's your world you live in. You have more power than you know.

Breathe deeply and simply 'be' now. Face your fears. Take responsibility. Change comes from making better choices. Learn from your past and let it go.
Your life matters. You are important. Value and love yourself unconditionally. Squeeze the joy. Live with passion. Feel alive. Have no regrets.
Surround yourself with those who believe in you. Show gratitude in abundance. Fill your life with what excites you. You deserve to fly high.
Expand your ways of thinking. Throw off old beliefs that don't serve you. Life's not meant to be a treadmill. You are not on this earth to simply 'exist'.

Give up your excuses.
Stop waiting to be rescued.
Limitations exist in your mind only.

All change begins with YOU.

For more information visit **maureensharphouse.com**

ENDNOTES

1   Goldberg, Daniel S, and Summer J McGee, "Pain as a Global Public Health Priority," *BMC Public Health* 11, no, 1 (2011), https://doi.org/10.1186/1471-2458-11-770.

2   Zelaya, Carla E., James M. Dahlhamer, Jacqueline W. Lucas, and Eric M. Connor, "Chronic Pain and High-Impact Chronic Pain Among U.S. Adults, 2019," NCHS Data Brief, no 390, Hyattsville, MD: National Center for Health Statistics, 2020, https://www.cdc.gov/nchs/products/databriefs/db390.htm.

3   Breivik, Harald, Beverly Collett, Vittorio Ventafridda, Rob Cohen, and Derek Gallacher, "Survey of Chronic Pain in Europe: Prevalence, Impact on Daily Life, and Treatment," *European Journal of Pain* 10, no, 4 (2006): 287–87, https://doi.org/10.1016/j.ejpain.2005.06.009.

4   "Media Resources," *British Pain Society*, Accessed October 9, 2021, https://www.britishpainsociety.org/media-resources/.

5   According to Burning Nights CRPS, 'The McGill Pain Index is a scale that shows the rating or level of pain. It was originally developed as the McGill pain questionnaire back in 1971 at the McGill University by two researchers; Ronald Melzack and Warren Togerson.

"Pain Scale," *Burning Nights CRPS*, November 12, 2020, https://www.burningnightscrps.org/sufferers/pain-scale/.

6   "Thought (Disambiguation)," *Wikipedia*, Wikimedia Foundation, August 19, 2019, https://en.wikipedia.org/wiki/Thought_(disambiguation).

7   "Hope," *Wikipedia*, Wikimedia Foundation, September 30, 2021, https://en.wikipedia.org/wiki/Hope.

8   Pruett, Barbara J., *Marty Robbins: Fast Cars and Country Music*, Scarecrow Press, 2007.

9   "Ben Greenhalgh Quote," *AZquotes*, Accessed October 10, 2021, https://www.azquotes.com/quote/811867.

10 "Self-Care: Taking Care of Your Body," *The Summit Counseling Center*, August 8, 2020, https://summitcounseling.org/self-care-taking-care-of-your-body/.

11 Shell, Marc, *Polio and Its Aftermath: The Paralysis of Culture*, Harvard University Press, 2009.

12 Moeller, Kristen, *What Are You Waiting For?: Learn How to Rise to the Occasion of Your Life*, Start Publishing LLC, 2013.

13 Freewheeling4, "'Creating the Spectacle!' Online - Part 1 - Finding Freedom.," YouTube Video, 4:43, August 17, 2012, https://www.youtube.com/watch?v=IPh533ht5AU.

DEFINITION SOURCES

American Heritage® Dictionary of the English Language, Fifth Edition from https://www.thefreedictionary.com/.

Cambridge Dictionary. https://dictionary.cambridge.org/.

Definitions.net, STANDS4 LLC, 2021. https://www.definitions.net/

Dictionary.com. https://www.dictionary.com/.

Farlex Dictionary of Idioms from https://idioms.thefree dictionary.com/.

Lexico Dictionaries | English. https://www.lexico.com/uk-english.

Longman Dictionary of Contemporary English Online. https://www.ldoceonline.com/.

Macmillan Dictionary. https://www.macmillandictionary.com/.

Merriam-Webster. https://www.merriam-webster.com/.

Oxford Learner's Dictionaries. https://www.oxford learnersdictionaries.com/us/definition/english/.

Oxford Reference. https://www.oxfordreference.com/.

Princeton's WordNet. https://wordnet.princeton.edu/

Theopedia.com. https://www.theopedia.com/.

Urban Dictionary. https://www.urbandictionary.com/.

Vocabulary.com. Vocabulary.com, Inc.
https://www.vocabulary.com/dictionary/.

Wiktionary. https://en.wiktionary.org/.

WordWeb Online Dictionary and Thesaurus.
https://www.wordwebonline.com/.

YourDictionary. https://www.yourdictionary.com/.

ABOUT THE AUTHOR

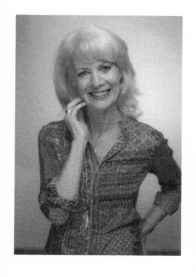

Maureen Sharphouse lives with her husband, Peter, and their dog, Jackson, in the village of Milnathort, Kinross-shire, Scotland. She is a coach, mentor, writer, and speaker. Maureen's passion is to inspire and help individuals live a unique legacy they are proud of. Her mission is to help people discover who they are beyond their physical body, live their best lives, and restore and unleash their soul's fire and passion. Maureen's vibrant enthusiasm for life is evident despite living with severe daily pain and complex ongoing health challenges. She is a lover of morning sunrises, good coffee, fresh flowers in her home, and spending time with her much-loved family and grandchildren.

You can connect with Maureen at MaureenSharphouse.com.

Maureen
Sharphouse.

YOUR NEXT BEST STEPS:

Reach out to me if you feel you would benefit from further support. If you need help navigating the often-challenging path of pain and illness, I am here for you. We can connect no matter where you live in the world. For a daily dose of uplifting words of wisdom and affirmations, you can connect with me on Facebook at *Facebook.com/MaureenSharphouse.Coaching*. If you would like to enquire about my personal mentoring or one-to-one coaching, the Unhackable Soul online course (based on the content of this book), or workshops and speaking engagements, you can email me directly at *Maureen@MaureenSharphouse.com*. The bottom line is, please reach out. I'd love to come alongside you to help reignite fire into your soul so you can live a life fuelled by joy, enthusiasm, and purpose.

ONE SIMPLE REQUEST

Now that you have discovered *Unhackable Soul*, I leave you with one simple request. If what I shared with you in this book has made a positive difference to you in some way, please spread and share the message. Living with pain and illness is far from easy, but it should never stop you from fully embracing life and stepping into your unique role in this world. Please tell people about *Unhackable Soul*. Gift them a copy of the book if you can or point them in the direction of my Facebook page or website. No one suffering chronic pain should have to withdraw to the side-lines of life and feel unsupported or alone.

YOU'VE READ THE BOOK

Ready to dive deeper and take the 30-day online course?
Stop retreating from life. Choose to *rise*.
It's time to restore life to your spirit and
soul and become Unhackable.

Start your 30-day journey today.
Visit MaureenSharphouse.com/unhackable-soul

UNHACKABLE SOULS TOGETHER

By coming together and supporting one another, we can all stay strong.

I invite you to visit my website to access my free downloadable guided meditation audio recordings, blog posts, and further personal development resources.

Visit MaureenSharphouse.com

FOR MEDIA, SPEAKING, AND WORKSHOP ENQUIRIES

Whether your audience is big or small and whatever your media, speaking, or workshop requirements, I will be happy to speak with you and explore how I can help you create a memorable and impacting event.

Email me directly at Maureen@MaureenSharphouse.com

BECOME A CERTIFIED
UNHACKABLE COACH

Get Paid to Help People Close their Gaps
Between Dreaming and Doing

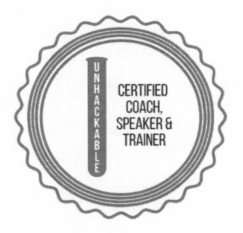

Learn More
https://bitly.com/unhackablesoulmc

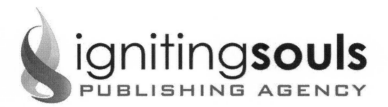

ignitingsouls
PUBLISHING AGENCY

Our mission is to help authors, coaches, entrepreneurs, and speakers write, publish, and market their books the right way—and turn them into eighteen streams of income.

You have a message to share and an audience to serve.

Let us do everything else. Chat with our team today to learn how we can help.

IgnitingSouls.com/apply

Made in the USA
Middletown, DE
10 May 2022

65570502R00168